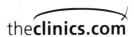

theclinics.com

MEDICAL CLINICS
OF NORTH AMERICA

Bariatric Surgery Primer
for the Internist

GUEST EDITORS
Nilesh A. Patel, MD
Lisa S. Koche, MD

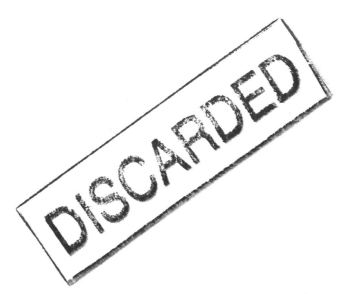

May 2007 • Volume 91 • Number 3

SAUNDERS

An Imprint of Elsevier, Inc.
PHILADELPHIA LONDON TORONTO MONTREAL SYDNEY TOKYO

W.B. SAUNDERS COMPANY
A Division of Elsevier Inc.

1600 John F. Kennedy Boulevard • Suite 1800 • Philadelphia, Pennsylvania 19103-2899

http://www.theclinics.com

MEDICAL CLINICS OF NORTH AMERICA
May 2007
Editor: Rachel Glover

Volume 91, Number
ISSN 0025-71
ISBN-13: 978-1-4160-498
ISBN-10: 1-4160-4986

The ideas and opinions expressed in *Medical Clinics of North America* do not necessarily reflect those of t Publisher. The Publisher does not assume any responsibility for any injury and/or damage to persons property arising out of or related to any use of the material contained in this periodical. The reader is a vised to check the appropriate medical literature and the product information currently provided by t manufacturer of each drug to be administered to verify the dosage, the method and duration of admini tration, or contraindications. It is the responsibility of the treating physician or other health care profe sional, relying on independent experience and knowledge of the patient, to determine drug dosages ar the best treatment for the patient. Mention of any product in this issue should not be construed as endors ment by the contributors, editors, or the Publisher of the product or manufacturers' claims.

Medical Clinics of North America (ISSN 0025-7125) is published bimonthly by W.B. Saunders, 360 Park Aven South, New York, NY 10010-1710. Business and editorial offices: 1600 John F. Kennedy Boulevard, Suite 180 Philadelphia, PA 19103-2899. Accounting and circulation offices: 6277 Sea Harbor Drive, Orlando, FL 3288 4800. Periodicals postage paid at New York, NY, and additional mailing offices. Subscription prices are US 157 per year for US individuals, USD 273 per year for US institutions, USD 81 per year for US students, US 200 per year for Canadian individuals, USD 347 per year for Canadian institutions, USD 119 per year f Canadian students, USD 227 per year for international individuals, USD 347 per year for international instit tions and USD 119 per year for international students. To receive student/resident rate, orders must be accor panied by name of affiliated institution, date of term, and the *signature* of program/residency coordinator c institution letterhead. Orders will be billed at individual rate until proof of status is received. Foreign air spee delivery is included in all *Clinics* subscription prices. All prices are subject to change without notic POSTMASTER: Send address changes to *Medical Clinics of North America*, Elsevier Periodicals Customer Se vice, 6277 Sea Harbor Drive, Orlando, FL 32887-4800. **Customer Service: 1-800-654-2452 (US). From outsic of the USA, call (+1) 407-345-1000. E-mail: hhspcs@harcourt.com.**

Reprints. For copies of 100 or more, of articles in this publication, please contact the Commercial Reprin Department, Elsevier Inc., 360 Park Avenue South, New York, New York 10010-1710. Tel.: (+1) (212) 63 3813; Fax: (+1) (212) 462-1935; E-mail: reprints@elsevier.com.

Medical Clinics of North America is also published in Spanish by McGraw-Hill Interamericana Editores S. A P.O. Box 5-237, 06500 Mexico, D.F., Mexico.

Medical Clinics of North America is covered in *Index Medicus, Current Contents, ASCA, Excerpta Medic Science Citation Index,* and *ISI/BIOMED.*

Printed in the United States of America.

GOAL STATEMENT

The goal of *Medical Clinics of North America* is to keep practicing physicians up to date with current clinical practice by providing timely articles reviewing the state of the art in patient care.

ACCREDITATION

The *Medical Clinics of North America* is planned and implemented in accordance with the Essential Areas and Policies of the Accreditation Council for Continuing Medical Education (ACCME) through the joint sponsorship of the University of Virginia School of Medicine and Elsevier. The University of Virginia School of Medicine is accredited by the ACCME to provide continuing medical education for physicians.

The University of Virginia School of Medicine designates this educational activity for a maximum of 90 *AMA PRA Category 1 Credits*™. Physicians should only claim credit commensurate with the extent of their participation in the activity.

The American Medical Association has determined that physicians not licensed in the US who participate in this CME activity are eligible for *AMA PRA Category 1 Credits*™.

Credit can be earned by reading the text material, taking the CME examination online at http://www.theclinics.com/home/cme, and completing the evaluation. After taking the test, you will be required to review any and all incorrect answers. Following completion of the test and evaluation, your credit will be awarded and you may print your certificate.

FACULTY DISCLOSURE/CONFLICT OF INTEREST

The University of Virginia School of Medicine, as an ACCME accredited provider, endorses and strives to comply with the Accreditation Council for Continuing Medical Education (ACCME) Standards of Commercial Support, Commonwealth of Virginia statutes, University of Virginia policies and procedures, and associated federal and private regulations and guidelines on the need for disclosure and monitoring of proprietary and financial interests that may affect the scientific integrity and balance of content delivered in continuing medical education activities under our auspices.

The University of Virginia School of Medicine requires that all CME activities accredited through this institution be developed independently and be scientifically rigorous, balanced and objective in the presentation/discussion of its content, theories and practices.

All authors/editors participating in an accredited CME activity are expected to disclose to the readers relevant financial relationships with commercial entities occurring within the past 12 months (such as grants or research support, employee, consultant, stock holder, member of speakers bureau, etc.). The University of Virginia School of Medicine will employ appropriate mechanisms to resolve potential conflicts of interest to maintain the standards of fair and balanced education to the reader. Questions about specific strategies can be directed to the Office of Continuing Medical Education, University of Virginia School of Medicine, Charlottesville, Virginia.

The authors/editors listed below have identified no professional or financial affiliations for themselves or their spouse/ partner:
Garth Davis, MD; Emmanuel Esaka, MD, PhD; Franco Folli, MD, PhD; Rachel Glover (Acquisitions Editor); Daniel B. Jones, MD, MS, FACS; LaShanda Jones, PhD; Todd A. Kellogg, MD; Lisa S. Koche, MD (Guest Editor); Rajesh Kuruba, MD; Daniel B. Leslie, MD; Troy A. Markel, MD; Nilesh A. Patel, MD (Guest Editor); Jitesh A. Patel, MD; Antonio E. Pontiroli, MD; Kinga A. Powers, MD; Ramesh C. Ramanathan, MD, FRCS; Scott T. Rehrig, MD, LTC; Wayne H. Schwesinger, MD; Rebecca Stack, BA; Samuel Szomstein, MD, FACS; Ronald Thomas, MD; Olga N. Tucker, MD, FRCSI; Kent R. Van Sickle, MD; Thomas A. Wadden, PhD; and Noel S. Williams, MD.

The authors/editors listed below identified the following professional or financial affiliations for themselves or their spouse/partner:
Jeff W. Allen, MD is a consultant for Allergan/Inamed, Ethican Endo-Surgery, Autosuture, and Karl Storz.
Joseph J. Colella, MD received remuneration from Tyco-Auto Suture for teaching laproscopic technique to another physician.
Anthony N. Fabricatore, PhD is a consultant for Pfizer.
Daniel J. Gagne, MD has a Resident Educational Grant from US Surgical Corporation to provide resident surgical training.
Sayeed Ikramuddin, MD is on the speaker's bureau for Pfizer.
Peter Lopez, MD is on the speaker's bureau for Pfizer.
Michel A. Mathier, MD serves as a consultant for Actelion and Gilead, and is on the speaker's bureau for Actelion, Encylive, and GlaxoSmithKline.
Samer G. Mattar, MD received honorarium for a lecture for US Surgical.
Michel M. Murr, MD, FACS is a consultant for Tyco Healthcare Group, LP, and Sanofi Aventis.
Raul J. Rosenthal, MD, FACS has a research grant with, and serves as a consultant for, Ethicon Endosurgery and Synovis; and, has a research grant with Karl Storz Endoscopy.
David B. Sarwer, PhD is a consultant for Allergan; is a principle investigator in two studies for the National Institute of Diabetes and Digestive and Kidney Diseases.

Disclosure of Discussion of non-FDA approved uses for pharmaceutical products and/or medical devices:
The University of Virginia School of Medicine, as an ACCME provider, requires that all faculty presenters identify and disclose any "off label" uses for pharmaceutical and medical device products. The University of Virginia School of Medicine recommends that each physician fully review all the available data on new products or procedures prior to instituting them with patients.

TO ENROLL

To enroll in the Medical Clinics of North America Continuing Medical Education program, call customer service at 1-800-654-2452 or visit us online at http://www.theclinics.com/home/cme. The CME program is available to subscribers for an additional fee of USD 205.

FORTHCOMING ISSUES

RECENT ISSUES

THE CLINICS ARE NOW AVAILABLE ONLINE!

Access your subscription at:
http://www.theclinics.com

GUEST EDITORS

NILESH A. PATEL, MD, Associate Director of Bariatric Surgery, Clinical Assistant Professor, Department of Surgery, University of Texas Health Science Center, San Antonio, Texas

LISA S. KOCHE, MD, Director, Spectra Complete Healthcare, Florida Cardiovascular Institute; Assistant Professor of Internal Medicine, University of South Florida; Weight Management and Metabolic Health Center, Tampa, Florida

CONTRIBUTORS

JEFF W. ALLEN, MD, Associate Professor of Surgery, Associate Professor, Department of Surgery, University of Louisville, Louisville, Kentucky

JOSEPH J. COLELLA, MD, Assistant Professor, Department of Surgery, Drexel University College of Medicine, Philadelphia; Director, Division of Bariatric Surgery, Department of Surgery, Allegheny General Hospital, Pittsburgh, Pennsylvania

GARTH DAVIS, MD, Houston Surgical Consultants, Houston, Texas

EMMANUEL ESAKA, MD, PhD, Resident in Obstetrics and Gynecology, Department of Obstetrics and Gynecology, Allegheny General Hospital, Pittsburgh, Pennsylvania

ANTHONY N. FABRICATORE, PhD, Assistant Professor, Department of Psychiatry, University of Pennsylvania School of Medicine, Philadelphia, Pennsylvania

FRANCO FOLLI, MD, PhD, Associate Professor, Director of Metabolic and Molecular Research, Department of Medicine, Diabetes Division, University of Texas Health Science Center, San Antonio, Texas

DANIEL J. GAGNE, MD, Director, Minimally Invasive Surgery Program, Department of Surgery, The Western Pennsylvania Hospital; Clinical Associate Professor, Surgery, Temple University, Pittsburgh, Pennsylvania

SAYEED IKRAMUDDIN, MD, Associate Professor, Section of Gastrointestinal Surgery, Department of Surgery, University of Minnesota, Minneapolis, Minnesota

DANIEL B. JONES, MD, MS, FACS, Associate Professor, Harvard Medical School; Chief, Section of Minimally Invasive Surgery, Beth Israel Deaconess Medical Center, Boston, Massachusetts

LASHANDA JONES, PhD, Postdoctoral Researcher, Department of Psychiatry, University of Pennsylvania School of Medicine, Philadelphia, Pennsylvania

TODD A. KELLOGG, MD, Assistant Professor, Section of Gastrointestinal Surgery, Department of Surgery, University of Minnesota, Minneapolis, Minnesota

LISA S. KOCHE, MD, Director, Spectra Complete Healthcare, Florida Cardiovascular Institute; Assistant Professor of Internal Medicine, University of South Florida; Weight Management and Metabolic Health Center, Tampa, Florida

RAJESH KURUBA, MD, Fellow, Advanced Laparoscopic GI and Bariatric Surgery, Department of Bariatric Surgery, University of South Florida, c/o Tampa General Hospital; Weight Management and Metabolic Health Center, Tampa, Florida

DANIEL LESLIE, MD, Surgical Fellow, Section of Gastrointestinal Surgery, Department of Surgery, University of Minnesota, Minneapolis, Minnesota

PETER P. LOPEZ, MD, Assistant Professor, Department of Surgery, University of Texas Health Science Center, San Antonio, Texas

TROY A. MARKEL, MD, Department of Surgery, Indiana University School of Medicine, Indianapolis, Indiana

MICHAEL A. MATHIER, MD, Assistant Professor of Medicine, Heart Failure/Transplantation, University of Pittsburgh School of Medicine; Director, Pulmonary Hypertension Program; Director, Cardiovascular Fellowship Program, Pittsburgh, Pennsylvania

SAMER G. MATTAR, MD, Director, Clarian Bariatric Center; Associate Professor, Department of Surgery, Indiana University School of Medicine, Indianapolis, Indiana

MICHEL M. MURR, MD, FACS, Director of Bariatric Surgery; Associate Professor of Surgery, Department of Bariatric Surgery, University of South Florida, c/o Tampa General Hospital; Weight Management and Metabolic Health Center, Tampa, Florida

JITESH A. PATEL, MD, Resident in General Surgery, Department of Surgery, Allegheny General Hospital, Pittsburgh, Pennsylvania

NILESH A. PATEL, MD, Associate Director of Bariatric Surgery, Clinical Assistant Professor, Department of Surgery, University of Texas Health Science Center, San Antonio, Texas

ANTONIO E. PONTIROLI, MD, Professor of Internal Medicine, Department of Medicine, University of Milano, Ospedale San Paolo, Milano, Italy

KINGA A. POWERS, MD, Minimally Invasive Surgery Fellow, Harvard Medical School, Beth Israel Deaconess Medical Center, Boston, Massachusetts

RAMESH C. RAMANATHAN, MD, FRCS, Assistant Professor of Surgery, Minimally Invasive and Bariatric Surgery, University of Pittsburgh School of Medicine, Pittsburgh, Pennsylvania

SCOTT T. REHRIG, MD, LTC, Minimally Invasive Surgery Fellow, Harvard Medical School, Beth Israel Deaconess Medical Center, Boston, Massachusetts

RAUL J. ROSENTHAL, MD, FACS, The Bariatric Institute, Cleveland Clinic Florida, Weston, Florida

DAVID B. SARWER, PhD, Associate Professor, Department of Psychiatry; Department of Surgery, University of Pennsylvania School of Medicine, Philadelphia, Pennsylvania

WAYNE H. SCHWESINGER, MD, Professor of Surgery, Department of Surgery, University of Texas Health Science Center, San Antonio, Texas

REBECCA STACK, BA, Research Coordinator, Department of Psychiatry, University of Pennsylvania School of Medicine, Philadelphia, Pennsylvania

SAMUEL SZOMSTEIN, MD, FACS, The Bariatric Institute, Cleveland Clinic Florida, Weston, Florida

RONALD L. THOMAS, MD, Associate Professor, Department of Obstetrics and Gynecology, Drexel University College of Medicine, Philadelphia; Director, Division of Maternal/Fetal Medicine, Division of Obstetrics and Gynecology, Allegheny General Hospital, Pittsburgh, Pennsylvania

OLGA N. TUCKER, MD, FRCSI, The Bariatric Institute, Cleveland Clinic Florida, Weston, Florida

KENT R. VAN SICKLE, MD, Assistant Professor of Surgery, Division of General and Laparoendoscopic Surgery, University of Texas Health Science Center San Antonio, San Antonio, Texas

THOMAS A. WADDEN, PhD, Professor, Department of Psychiatry, University of Pennsylvania School of Medicine, Philadelphia, Pennsylvania

NOEL S. WILLIAMS, MD, Assistant Professor, Department of Surgery, University of Pennsylvania School of Medicine, Philadelphia, Pennsylvania

CONTENTS

Obesity constitutes a major health problem with serious social and economic consequences worldwide. In North America, nearly one third of the population is obese, and this figure includes children and adolescents who are likely to become obese adults. Obesity carries a great financial impact on society; consequently, treating morbidly obese patients with surgery may offer substantial economic savings. This article summarizes the financial burdens of obesity and the economics of treating obesity in North America. It addresses the medical effectiveness and cost-effectiveness of bariatric surgery and the new regulations and accreditations for bariatric surgery programs.

The prevalence of morbid obesity in the United States and world-wide is increasing at an alarming rate. The number of bariatric surgical procedures also has steadily increased during the past decade. This article reviews the published literature and current practice trends for preoperative workup and assessment of patients undergoing bariatric surgery.

at risk for, or already suffering from, cardiovascular disease. Weight loss induced by the surgery has been shown to improve cardiovascular risk factors, cardiac structure and function, and the clinical course of established cardiovascular disease. The role of adipocyte-derived cytokines in mediating cardiovascular pathophysiology in obesity-and its modulation after weight loss-is under active investigation.

surgery and describes changes in functioning that can be expected with surgically induced weight loss. The article combines a review of the literature with clinical impressions gained from the more than 2500 candidates for bariatric surgery whom the authors have evaluated at the Hospital of the University of Pennsylvania.

Practitioners taking care of postoperative bariatric patients need to keep in mind all of the complications that this population faces to prevent unnecessary morbidity. Bariatric patients presenting postoperatively with abdominal pain, tachycardia, vomiting, tachypnea, and a sense of impending doom should be worked up aggressively to find the cause of their symptoms. Because the incidence of obesity is rising in children and adults, more patients will have surgery to help with their weight loss. Physicians caring for these patients must be able to diagnosis and treat their complications quickly and efficiently to prevent further complications.

Weight loss surgery, also known as bariatric surgery, has evolved from a specialty dominated by intestinal bypasses and vertical banded gastroplasty to its current state of a specialty characterized by minimal access techniques and Centers of Excellence. Bariatric surgery has remained the only reliably effective option for significant weight loss for the morbidly obese. This article reviews common problems occurring after laparoscopic adjustable gastric band with emphasis on conservative diagnosis and effective treatment.

Nutritional deficiencies are already present in many morbidly obese patients before weight-loss surgery. Appropriate preoperative detection and correction is essential. The severity and pattern of deficiencies is dependent on the presence of preoperative uncorrected deficiency, the type of procedure performed varying with the degree of restriction or the length of bypassed small intestine, the modification of eating behavior, the development of complications, compliance with oral multivitamin and mineral supplementation, and compliance with follow-up. Rigorous control of fluids and electrolytes with establishment of adequate oral nutrition is important in the immediate postoperative period. Regular follow-up of the metabolic and nutritional status of the patient is essential, with life-long multivitamin and mineral supplementation.

ELSEVIER
SAUNDERS

Med Clin N Am 91 (2007) xv–xvi

THE MEDICAL
CLINICS
OF NORTH AMERICA

Preface

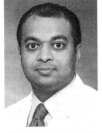 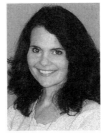

Nilesh A. Patel, MD   Lisa S. Koche, MD
Guest Editors

Obesity has reached epidemic proportions among most industrialized countries in the world, and unfortunately the United States continues to be a world leader. The impact of obesity on this country's economy and health care system will be accentuated as obesity quickly becomes the number-one cause of preventable death in the United States.

The National Care Determination released in February 2006 was a landmark development in the treatment of morbid obesity (http://www.cms.hhs.gov/transmittals/downloads/R54NCD.pdf). Within this determination, surgery was defined as the true "standard of care" for morbid obesity, opening access to care for Medicare recipients. Most experts feel that this determination will strongly influence medical policy among private payers nationwide.

At the same time, the National Care Determination placed a relative limit on access to care as weight-loss procedures were restricted to designated "centers of excellence." We all hope that this restriction to access is short lived as the number of designated centers increases. The intangible positive that has come from the limitation to access is the clear and intuitive need for primary care physicians, internists, and medical subspecialists to work cohesively as a team with surgeons in the management, treatment, and prevention of morbid obesity.

The decision for Elsevier to invite a surgeon teamed with a medical specialist to organize and present this volume is a tremendous step in formulating this much-needed multidisciplinary alliance against obesity. By creating this volume, we hope to achieve three primary objectives.

doi:10.1016/j.mcna.2007.03.002   *medical.theclinics.com*

The first and foremost objective is to put in perspective the impact of obesity on the American economy and the significant health risks related to obesity. The next objective is to delineate the rationale for surgery and the role of the internist in this undertaking. This is a critical point as the internist will continue to have a pivotal role in identifying a surgical candidate, directing a consultation to an appropriate surgeon, assessing outcomes, and identifying known complications of the most common procedures. Lastly, this volume provides a comprehensive summary of the impact of surgery on known comorbidities associated with obesity. In achieving these goals, we have been able to show the value of a much-needed multidisciplinary team approach.

The editors would like to thank all of the contributors to this volume. Its comprehensive overview would not have been possible without their much appreciated effort. In addition, we would like to thank Rachel Glover, Editor for the *Medical Clinics of North America*, for giving us the distinguished opportunity to serve as her Guest Editors for this unique volume. We hope we have lived up to her insightful vision for this volume as it was truly an honor to serve as her Guest Editors.

Nilesh A. Patel, MD
Department of Surgery
University of Texas Health Science Center San Antonio
7703 Floyd Curl Drive, MC7740
San Antonio, TX 78229, USA

E-mail address: drpatel@bypassdoc.com

Lisa S. Koche, MD
Internal Medicine
University of South Florida
509 South Armenia Avenue
Suite #302
Tampa, FL 33609, USA

E-mail address: LKOCHE@fciheart.com

ELSEVIER
SAUNDERS

THE MEDICAL
CLINICS
OF NORTH AMERICA

Med Clin N Am 91 (2007) xvii

Dedication

The Guest Editors would like to dedicate this issue of the *Medical Clinics of North America* to our families. Without their support and patience throughout the publication process, this issue would not have been possible.

Thank you to my wife, Hemal, and my daughter, Nitya.
  Nilesh A. Patel, MD
Thank you to my husband, David, and my daughter, Jordyn.
  Lisa S. Koche, MD

THE MEDICAL
CLINICS
OF NORTH AMERICA

ELSEVIER
SAUNDERS

Med Clin N Am 91 (2007) 321–338

Financial Impact of Obesity and Bariatric Surgery

Kinga A. Powers, MD, Scott T. Rehrig, MD,
Daniel B. Jones, MD, MS, FACS*

*Harvard Medical School, Beth Israel Deaconess Medical Center,
330 Brookline Avenue, Boston, MA 02215, USA*

Obesity constitutes a major health problem with serious social and economic consequences worldwide. According to the World Health Organization (WHO), obesity has become a "global epidemic" affecting more people than hunger [1]. In North America, nearly one third of the population is obese, and this figure includes children and adolescents who are likely to become obese adults. Obesity is a major avoidable risk factor for noncommunicable diseases and poses a great risk for higher all-cause mortality at any age. Bariatric surgery is an important treatment option that is effective at weight reduction and has been shown to improve quality of life. Bariatric surgery cures many comorbidities of morbid obesity, such as diabetes, hypertension, and dyslipidemias, which are associated with increased mortality and health costs. Obesity carries a great financial impact on society; consequently, treating morbidly obese patients with surgery may offer substantial economic savings. Therefore, physicians caring for obese patients should be familiar with the basic health economics that dictate funding and policy for treatments of this increasingly prevalent disease. This article summarizes the financial burdens of obesity and the economics of treating obesity in North America. It addresses the medical effectiveness and cost-effectiveness of bariatric surgery and the new regulations and accreditations for bariatric surgery programs.

Obesity and its risks

Body mass index (BMI), calculated as weight in kilograms divided by height in meters^2, is the most commonly used tool to evaluate a patient's

---

* Corresponding author. Beth Israel Deaconess Medical Center, 330 Brookline Avenue, Boston, MA 02215.
E-mail address: Djones1@BIDMC.Harvard.edu (D.B. Jones).

weight status. An individual is defined as being overweight with a BMI of 25 to 29.9, obesity is defined as a BMI of 30 to 39.9, and morbid obesity is defined as a BMI of 40 or greater (or 35 in the presence of comorbidities). Comorbidities depend on the degree of obesity and include diabetes, hypertension, dyslipidemia, obstructive sleep apnea, weight-related arthropathies, stress urinary incontinence, depression, and cancer (breast, uterus, prostate, and colon) [2]. People who have a BMI greater than 30 have a 50% higher risk of dying than those who have a healthy BMI. A BMI greater than 30 is associated with a higher all-cause mortality even after adjusting for potential confounding factors at any age [3–5]. Evidence suggests that bariatric surgery ameliorates the risk of dying from obesity-related diseases. In a retrospective study, Flum and Dellinger [6] demonstrated that at 1 year after bariatric surgery, the adjusted hazard for death was 33% lower than that of patients who did not undergo bariatric surgery. In the same study, for patients younger than 40 years of age, mortality by 14 years post-bariatric surgery was reported at 3%, compared with 13% without the procedure [6]. In another study, gastric bypass reduced the relative risk of death by 89% [7].

Prevalence of obesity

Current estimates are that there are over 300 million obese people worldwide, which is a substantial increase from the estimated 200 million 10 years ago [8]. In the United States, nearly two thirds of the adult population is overweight (including those who are obese), and one third of the adult population is obese. The most recent U.S. National Health and Nutrition Examination Survey (NHANES) report compared the age-adjusted prevalence of overweight and obese United States adults 20 to 75 years of age. Their figures demonstrated that from 1976 to 2004, the percentage of overweight and obese adults increased from 47.0% to 66.3% (Fig. 1). Obesity more than doubled during this period (from 15.0% to 32.9%). The increase in obesity was more common in men than in women: Between 1999 and 2004, women's obesity rates did not change significantly (from 33.4% to 33.2%) [9].

This obesity epidemic is not limited to adults. According to the NHANES, from 1988 to 2004, the percentage of obese children 6 to 11 years of age grew from 11% to 19%. Among adolescents 12 to 19 years of age, the percentage of overweight individuals increased from 11% to 17% during the same period [10]. Studies show that these children are likely to become obese adults, further contributing to the obesity epidemic [11].

Canada is also facing an increase in obesity rates. According to statistics from Canada, in 2004, approximately 8.6 million (36.1%) Canadian adults 18 years of age and over were overweight; of those, 5.5 million were obese (23.1%) [12]. This is a dramatic increase from the estimated 14% obesity rate reported in 1978/1979. Obesity rates vary among the Canadian

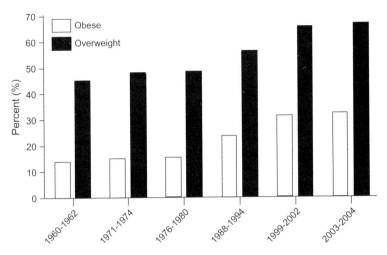

Fig. 1. Prevalence of overweight and obesity among adults 20 years of age and older in the United States, 2003–2004. Overweight is defined as BMI 25 to 29.9. Obesity is defined as BMI 30 and above. *Data from* National Center for Health Statistics Health, United States, 2005.

provinces, with the highest in Newfoundland and Labrador and the lowest in British Columbia. Similar to the United States, in Canada, obesity among children 2 to 17 years of age is on the rise, increasing from 3% in 1978/79 to 8% by 2004 [12].

Economic burden of obesity

As the average American waistline increases, so do obesity-related illnesses and, consequently, health care costs. Obesity causes worker productivity to suffer and shortens the number of productive life years due to increased mortality, which adds to the societal burden. The simplest way of classifying the considerable economic strain of obesity is to divide its expense into direct and indirect costs. Direct health care costs can be defined as those associated with diagnosing and treating disease, including physician reimbursement, cost of medications, and cost of hospital and home nursing services. Indirect costs relate to morbidity and mortality and are a reflection of lost wages because of illness or disability and of a loss of future earnings due to premature death.

The WHO estimates the total cost of obesity at 2% to 7% of total health care costs worldwide [13]. In the United States, the total (direct and indirect) cost of obesity treatment has been estimated at $117 billion in 2001 dollars, which is likely higher today [14]. The annual direct cost of caring for overweight and obese patients in the United States has been estimated at

$92.6 billion in 2002 dollars. According to a study by Finkelstein and colleagues [15], the total United States medical costs of overweight and obese patients accounted for 9.1% of total United States medical expenditures in 1998 and was thought to rival the medical expenditures attributable to smoking, which range between 6.5% and 14.4%. Across the United States, the state-level obesity medical expenditure estimates ranged from $87 million (Wyoming) to $7.7 billion (California) [15,16]. Obese adults have been shown to incur 37.4% greater annual medical expenditures than normal-weight persons. These expenditures ranged from 26.1% for out-of-pocket expenses to 36.8% for Medicare and 39.1% for Medicaid insurance expenses [15].

The direct costs of obesity represent a substantial cost comparable to the economic burden of other diseases, such as cancer. For example, in 2004, the costs related to cancer treatment in the United States were estimated at $72.1 billion, which translated to just less than 5% of total United States healthcare spending [17]. Although 84% of bariatric patients are women, it has been demonstrated that the groups that contribute most to the expense of treatment are morbidly obese men, specifically those with BMIs greater than 35 [18]. For example, in Illinois [19] the average annual cost of care in 2002 related to cardiovascular disease and diabetes was $12,342 for morbidly obese women and $13,674 for morbidly obese men.

Canadian obesity costs are not far behind United States costs. In Canada, the total cost of obesity was reported at $1.8 billion, corresponding to 2.4% of the total health care cost for all diseases in 1997, and increased to $4.3 billion in 2001 [20,21], with $1.6 billion in direct costs. Eighty percent of the total cost was due to treatment of comorbidities such as hypertension, noninsulin-dependent diabetes mellitus, and coronary artery disease.

The indirect cost is difficult to estimate but is projected at $58.8 billion worldwide and also rivals the economic burden of smoking [22]. In the United States, the indirect costs or the cost of lost productivity related to obesity among Americans 17 to 64 years of age has been estimated at $3.9 billion. This value can be broken down into 39.3 million workdays lost related to obesity, 62.7 million physician office visits, 239.0 million restricted activity days, and 89.5 million bed-days related to obesity [14]. Thompson and colleagues [23] calculated that obese men were absent 2.7 more days per year than ideal-weight men, and obese women missed 5.1 more days per year than ideal-weight women. Similarly, Finkelstein and colleagues [24] determined that the 9% of all full-time employees eligible for bariatric surgery attributed to two thirds of the costs of obesity in the United States (~$90 billion per year). Obese workers had 5.1 additional days of work loss and $2230 higher annual medical costs. In the most recent report, an economic model for New Mexico by Frezza and colleagues [25] describes the cost of obesity in terms of lost business output, employment, and income. Total labor income lost was nearly $200 million, with a loss of 7300 jobs, translating to loss in local tax revenues of over $48 million.

Although the increasingly high direct and indirect costs of obesity can be measured, there are additional intangible costs that must be considered and are more difficult to quantify. These costs include underachievement in school, discrimination at work, psychosocial problems, and an overall poorer quality of life. The Medical Outcomes Study Short-Form Health Survey demonstrated that obese patients showed statistically poorer scores on all 10 subtests than did the normal-weight population. These subtests evaluated such aspects of health as physical functioning, social functioning, mental health, and pain [26]. Overall obesity is a chronic and debilitating disease with great social and economic consequences worldwide.

Etiology and nonsurgical management of obesity

Why are Americans so overweight, and is there anything that can be done to stop this epidemic? The etiology of this chronic disease is multifactorial. Studies point to an imbalance between increased calorie intake and decreased calorie output as the main cause of obesity [27]. An average American consumes over 3500 calories per day, with snacks contributing to about 20% to 25% of total energy intake [27]. The increased calorie intake is attributed to falling food costs due to an expansion of the food supply and heavy food marketing. Decreased food prices combined with skyrocketing advertising rates of fast food, restaurant food, snacks, and sugar-sweetened soft-drinks have resulted in an increased consumption of saturated fats, sugars, and energy-dense foods [27]. Shin-Yi Chou and colleagues [28] reported that since the 1960s, American households doubled their food budget spent on restaurant meals, and 69% of the growth in the BMI of the American population can be attributed to the increase in the per capita number of restaurants. Increases in the price of cigarettes and restrictions on smoking have also been linked to trends in obesity [28]. The decline in calorie output has been hypothesized to result from technologic changes contributing to a reduction in daily physical activities. Additionally, more sedentary lifestyles with higher rates of passive rather then active entertainment is thought to contribute significantly to the rise in the North American obesity rates [29].

To help Americans lose weight, various behavioral therapies have emerged to address their changing lifestyles. These therapies focus on self-monitoring techniques, increasing exercise, stress management, cognitive restructuring, contingency management, and group support systems. Other nonsurgical methods include medications such as gastrointestinal lipase inhibitors, serotonin norepinephrine reuptake inhibitors, and appetite suppressants. Neither behavioral modification nor pharmacotherapy has been proven to have long-term sustainable results. A recent systematic review of nonsurgical weight loss programs revealed high costs, attrition rates, and the probability of regaining at least 50% of the lost weight in 1 to 2 years [3]. With medications such as fluoxetine, sibutramine, and orlistat, the magnitude of weight loss is less then 10 pounds at 1 year, and the long-term health benefits and risks remain unclear [30]. Even with modest weight loss, the rate of diabetes and hypertension may be reduced significantly; therefore, combining pharmacotherapy with behavioral therapy may be more successful [30]. Many new weight loss medications are being tested, and the demand for this type of therapy will likely increase in the future. Compared with surgery, the efficacy of commercially available self-help weight loss programs and prescription bariatric medications are inferior. Therefore, the role of nonsurgical means of weight loss and treating comorbidities in the obese population remains largely undefined.

Surgical options for obesity and their effectiveness

There are various bariatric surgical procedures that can be performed via open or laparoscopic surgery. These can be divided into malabsorptive (limiting nutrient absorption by bypassing parts of the gastrointestinal tract) and restrictive (decreasing the size of the stomach limiting food intake). Roux-en-Y gastric bypass (RYGB) is an example of a combined malabsorptive and restrictive procedure whereby the stomach is reduced to a small gastric pouch connected to a segment of jejunum downstream; this procedure bypasses the duodenum and proximal small intestine, reducing nutrient absorption. Vertical banded gastroplasty (VBG) and adjustable gastric banding (AGB) are restrictive techniques whereby the stomach is stapled or banded to create a small gastric pouch and a narrow gastric inlet that remains connected with the remainder of the stomach, thus reducing the volume ingested.

The morbidly obese population benefits from bariatric surgery when other means of weight loss, such as diet, increased exercise, behavioral therapy, and weight loss prescription drugs, have failed. In 1991, a National Institutes of Health Consensus Statement established the indications for bariatric surgery as morbid obesity (BMI > 40) or a BMI of at least 35 and serious comorbid conditions [31]. The benefits of surgery include weight loss, improvement in quality of life and comorbidities, and reduced relative risk of death.

A recent comprehensive review from Canada summarized data from 15 international systematic reviews available from the Cochrane and International Network of Agencies for Health Technology Assessment databases on the effectiveness of bariatric surgery (Tables 1 and 2) [32]. Malabsorptive procedures were demonstrated to be more efficacious at causing weight loss and eliminating comorbidities than restrictive procedures. Excess weight loss for RYGB ranged from 60% to 90%. The risks of mortality and adverse events were reported as higher than with the restrictive procedures.

A meta-analysis of 16,944 patients who had a baseline BMI of 46.85 reported a 62% excess weight loss for gastric bypass compared with 46% for AGB, 68% for gastroplasty, and 70% for biliopancreatic diversion/duodenal switch [33]. In most cases, weight loss was sustained at 2 years or more. The weakness of the meta-analysis was that it included randomized control

Table 1
Summary of findings on excess weight loss and resolution of comorbid conditions from Health Technology Assessments Review

Procedure	Excess weight loss,[a] range (%)	Resolution[b] of comorbid conditions, range (%)
Malabsorptive		
Roux-en-Y gastric bypass	60–90	Diabetes: 74–99
		Hypertension: 67–93
		Dyslipidemias: 73–99
Restrictive		
Adjustable gastric banding	42–60	Diabetes: 29–92
		Hypertension: 29–40
		Dyslipidemia: 24
Vertical banded gastroplasty	58–87	Diabetes: 100
		Hypertension: 50–60
		Dyslipidemias: 14–72

[a] Percentage of excess weight loss = (weight loss/excess weight) × 100 (where excess weight = total preoperative weight–ideal weight).
[b] Defined as the stopping of medication taken for comorbid condition.
From Medical Advisory Secretariat, Ontario Ministry of Health and Long-Term Care Government of Ontario. Bariatric Surgery Health Technology Literature Review, 2005; with permission.

trials with variable postsurgical follow-up ranging from 6 to 36 months. Nevertheless, the reduction of comorbid diseases was dramatic (Table 3). Diabetes resolved in 77%, hyperlipidemia resolved in 70%, and hypertension resolved in 62% of patients. Given that the annual costs of diabetes is estimated at $10,683, gastric bypass is cost effective even if only the diabetes is resolved [34].

Evidence from a prospective Swedish Obese Subjects (SOS) study indicates that sustained weight loss of 16% of Excess Body Weight (EBW) is achievable after bariatric surgery. After 2 years, weight had increased by 0.1% in the control group and had decreased by 23.4% in the surgical group. After 10 years, the weight of the control patients had risen by 1.6% (standard deviation [SD], 12%) from inclusion weight. The maintained weight change was −25%

Table 2
Summary of findings on mortality and adverse effects from Health Technology Assessments Review

Procedure	Mortality, range (%)	Adverse effects, range (%)
Malabsorptive		
Roux-en-Y gastric bypass	0.1–4.1	0.1–70
Restrictive		
Adjustable gastric banding	0–0.9	1.1–18
Vertical banded gastroplasty	0–0.8	1–30.4

From Medical Advisory Secretariat, Ontario Ministry of Health and Long-Term Care Government of Ontario. Bariatric Surgery Health Technology Literature Review, 2005; with permission.

Table 3
Outcomes for comorbid conditions after bariatric surgery

Type of surgery	Resolution of diabetes			Resolution of hypertension			Improvement in hyperlipidemia		
	Mean (%)	95% CI	n resolved/n evaluated	Mean (%)	95% CI	n resolved/n evaluated	Mean (%)	95% CI	n resolved/n evaluated
All types of bariatric surgery	76.8	70.7–82.9	1417/1846	61.7	55.6–67.8	3151/4805	79.3	88.2–90.5	846/1019
Roux-en-Y gastric bypass	83.7	77.3–90.1	829/989	67.5	58.4–76.5	1594/2115	96.9	93.6–100	117/125
Vertical banded gastroplasty	71.6	55.1–88.2	45/66	69.0	59.1–79.0	277/382	73.6	60.8–86.3	174/215
Other banding (fixed and variable)	47.9	29.1–66.7	98/205	43.2	30.4–55.9	232/604	58.9	28.2–89.6	333/426

Abbreviation: CI, confidence interval.

From Buchwald H, Avidor Y, Braunwald E, et al. Bariatric surgery: a systematic review and meta-analysis. JAMA 2004;292(14):1724–37; with permission. Copyright © 2004, American Medical Association. All rights reserved.

(SD, 11%) in the gastric bypass subgroup, −16.5% (SD, 11%) in the VBG subgroup, and −13.2% (SD, 13%) in the banding subgroup. At 8 years of follow-up, among 251 surgically treated patients, the average weight loss was 20 kg, whereas among 232 medically treated patients, the average weight did not change [35].

Studies have mostly considered open approaches; however, in the era of laparoscopic bariatric procedures, there is new evidence that the laparoscopic approach may offer some advantages. Puzziferri and colleagues [36] performed a randomized trial with a 3-year follow-up comparing laparoscopic gastric bypass with the open approach. He found that the rate of incisional hernia was significantly reduced and conferred a major advantage at long-term follow-up for the patients who underwent laparoscopic gastric bypass. The rate of cholecystectomy was greater after laparoscopic gastric bypass (28% versus 5%). Other studies comparing open versus laparoscopic gastric bypass report equal effectiveness with respect to weight loss, resolution of comorbidities, and quality of life improvement. Although laparoscopic surgery is on average a longer procedure than the open procedure, fewer serious complications were demonstrated. With laparoscopy, there was less blood loss, fewer intensive care unit admissions, and a shorter length of hospital stay [37]. In a recent outcomes study, mortality in the open group was 1.3 times that of the laparoscopic group [38]. The reoperative rate was greater after laparoscopic procedures [39]. Overall, laparoscopic is believed to be preferable to the open procedure; however, further randomized control trials are needed.

Bariatric surgery cost

Considering the exponential demand for bariatric surgery, it is essential to address its socioeconomic impact because limited health care resources in most countries may not be able to keep up with the obesity epidemic and increasing demands for effective treatment. In the United States, over 110,000 bariatric operations are performed each year. From 1998 to 2003, the number of bariatric operations increased by over 740% from 13,365 to 102,794, and the estimate is that in the year 2010, 218,000 operations will be performed [40]. Insurance coverage was distributed between privately insured patients accounting for 82%; Medicare, Medicaid, and self-pay accounting for 14% percent of surgeries; and other payers accounting for the remaining 3%. In 2002, Encinosa and colleagues [41] estimated that 11.5 million patients met clinical criteria for bariatric surgery; however, only 0.6% underwent surgery [42]. Because only a fraction of clinically eligible patients are treated surgically, potentially thousands of patients may not have access to appropriate surgical care.

Despite a decline in complication rates, hospital mortality rates, and length of stay for bariatric surgery patients, the cost of bariatric surgery has been increasing steadily. Hospital inpatient costs in the United States increased from $173 million in 1998 to $1.7 billion in 2003. The mean cost per operation for all payers increased 21% from $12,872 in 1998 to $15,533 in 2003, with the largest increase for Medicaide-covered procedures [43]. The Healthcare Cost and Utilization Project and the Agency for Healthcare Research and Quality tracks the costs of obesity surgery. In this database, inpatient costs for bariatric surgery were $16,541 in teaching hospitals and $14,406 in nonteaching hospitals. Rural hospitals were slightly more costly at $16,741, compared with urban hospitals at $15,447. Comparisons of average costs per patient demonstrated no cost savings in high-volume centers as compared with low-volume centers. Low-volume hospitals (<118 operations) had an average cost per patient of $16,402; high-volume hospitals (>387 operations) had average costs per patient of $16,339.

Gastric bypass is the most commonly performed procedure, accounting for 80% to 90% of bariatric surgeries, with gastroplasty decreasing from 24% to 7% in 2002 [40]. Laparoscopic gastric bypass was introduced in 1994; since then, an increasing number of weight loss surgeries have been performed laparoscopically and have achieved similar weight loss to open operations. Paxton and Matthews [44] examined the cost-effectiveness of the open (n = 6425) versus laparoscopic (n = 5867) procedures and demonstrated laparoscopic gastric bypass to be more cost effective, regardless of gender. On average, the total cost of laparoscopic RYGB was $17,660, compared with open gastric bypass costs of $20,443. Livingston [45] compared charges and noted laparoscopic gastric bypass costs at $19,794, open gastric bypass costs at $22,313, and laparoscopic adjustable gastric band costs at $25,355. The shorter length of stay for laparoscopic patients may not be financially advantageous to hospitals reimbursed on per diem basis [25].

Cost-effectiveness of bariatric surgery

As costs of obesity and its treatment continue to trend upward, policy makers must decide how best to spend limited healthcare dollars. Physicians need to understand the coverage criteria and remain actively involved in policy making for obese patients, especially for those who have failed multiple supervised diets, suffer comorbid conditions, and are considering bariatric surgery.

A number of studies have compared the cost-effectiveness and the cost benefit of bariatric operations with no treatment and with medical or behavioral treatment. A cost-effectiveness analysis (CEA) expresses the benefits of a procedure in nonmonetary terms, such as life-years gained or symptom-free days, whereas a cost-benefit analysis (CBA) places a specific dollar value on the years of life gained by a procedure. CEA is more applicable to medical treatments than CBA because CEA assesses quantity and quality of life generated by an intervention and is used more often by policy makers to prioritize resources. Cost-effectiveness is usually expressed as a cost in dollars per quality-adjusted life-years (QALY), or the cost-effectiveness ratio. The cost-effectiveness ratio is the ratio of change in costs to change in effects, such as increased QALY. A cost effectiveness ratio less than $50,000 is viewed as cost effective [46]. Some of the limitations of CEAs are as follows: (1) If an intervention is cost effective, it does not mean that it is inexpensive or that it represents a cost savings. Therefore, if health budgets are limited, even the most cost-effective procedures can be outweighed by competing interventions of even greater value. (2) CEA measures life-years saved or gained; however, CEA may not compare the same quality outcomes of those years and therefore may not be useful when comparing different areas of healthcare. Outcome measures used for various obesity treatments may be different, and a common currency must be applied when comparing them. Furthermore, studies using CEA often use different definitions of obesity and are short term. Consequently, CEA is an important criterion that can be used in developing health policy if it is interpreted with caution and as part of a number of other criteria that are beyond the scope of this review.

Are weight loss operations cost effective? Several studies have addressed this question and have found bariatric surgery to be cost effective when compared with no treatment or with pharmaceutical treatment alone. A number of studies applied CEA to determine the cost per QALY of surgery and reported results ranging from net savings of $4000 per QALY for vertical banded gastroplasty [47] to $35,600 per QALY for the gastric bypass procedure [48]. Van Gemert et al [47] studied a small cohort of 21 patients undergoing VBG and compared them with a hypothetical untreated cohort. This study considered the direct and indirect costs of obesity, including those related to comorbidities. The study concluded that surgical treatment saves $3928 to $4004 per QALY. This surgical procedure, although cost effective, is not commonly performed in the United States.

Craig and Tseng [48] analyzed cost effectiveness after open gastric bypass in men and women 35 to 55 years of age who had a BMI from 40 to 50 and who did not have cardiovascular disease and in whom conservative bariatric therapies had been unsuccessful. He found that although RYGB is not cost saving for the payer, it is cost effective for men and women compared with other interventions. Cost-effectiveness ratios ranged from $5000 to $16,000 per QALY for women and $10,000 to $35,600 per QALY for men, indicating that RYGB was more cost effective for women than for men. Furthermore, gastric bypass proved more cost effective for patients who had a BMI greater than 40 (Fig. 2) and less cost effective for older and less obese men [48]. In this study, there was no reduction in lifetime medical costs to patients; this lack of cost savings may be attributed to the patient selection for the study. Subjects did not have the chronic medical conditions typically associated with obesity, and several of their obesity-related indirect costs, such as decreased productivity and lost wages, were not included in the analysis.

In a systematic literature review from the United Kingdom, Clegg and colleagues [37] assessed weight change, quality of life, morbidity, mortality,

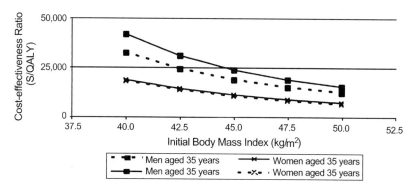

Fig. 2. Analysis of four risk subgroups representing the upper and lower bounds of the cost-effectiveness ratios. (*From* Craig BM, Tseng DS. Cost-effectiveness of gastric bypass for severe obesity. Am J Med 2002;113:491–8; with permission.)

revision rates, and obesity comorbidities in surgically versus nonsurgically treated obese patients. After 2 years, surgical patients had lost between 23 and 37 kg, and significant weight loss had been maintained up to 8 years after the surgery. Gastric bypass resulted in greater weight loss (6–14 kg more) and greater improvement in comorbid conditions compared with gastroplasty or jejunoileal bypass. All types of bariatric surgeries were shown to be cost effective when compared with nonsurgical management at £11,000 per QALY. Comparisons of the different types of surgery were reported as equivocal.

Two Canadian studies reported a CBA to determine the time frame for bariatric surgery to result in cost savings. Their data suggest that bariatric surgery becomes cost effective especially 2 to 3 years after the procedure [7,49]. In a two-cohort, 5-year study, patients who had RYGB (open or laparoscopic) or an open VBG (n = 1035) were compared with a nonsurgical obese group (n = 5,746). After 5 years, patients undergoing bariatric surgery had fewer hospitalizations and fewer physician visits, and the total direct health care cost was on average 45% higher for the control subjects. The cost per 1000 patients for hospitalizations was 29% higher for control subjects than for the bariatric surgery group. Data from these studies suggest that after 3.5 years, the initial investment for the weight-reduction surgery and related hospital care was compensated by a reduction in total costs of obesity treatment for these patients. The limitations of this study were no data on specific comorbidities and their outcomes and a poorly matched control group [50]. In contrast, a study from the United States by Finkelstein and colleagues [24] determined that it would likely take between 5 and 10 years for an employer to recover the full cost of the surgery unless an employee contributed a copay for the operation.

Bariatric surgery affects various components of healthcare that contribute to the cost of obesity (eg, the cost of medications after surgery). Several studies demonstrate that as the patient's comorbid conditions improve, the need for medications decreases, productivity increases, and therefore weight loss surgery can pay for itself within 3 years [51,52]. Snow and colleagues [52] estimated that the projected cost savings realized in their 78 patients were approximately $240,566.04 annually (Fig. 3). In contrast, using data from the SOS study, Narbro and colleagues [53] demonstrated that although surgical treatment lowered some medication costs (especially for diabetes mellitus and cardiovascular disease), it increased other medication costs, resulting in similar total costs for surgically and conventionally treated obese individuals at 6 years. The SOS intervention study was based on self-selected patients with data on medication use available for only 55% of the reference population; therefore, this may have affected the reliability of this study.

In summary, for morbidly obese people who have costly comorbid conditions, operative therapy offers a large potential benefit in quality of adjusted life-years and savings to the total medical expenses incurred by the patients and their employers.

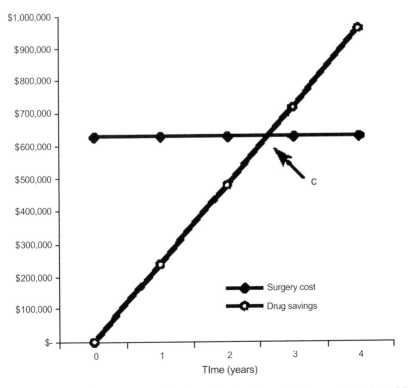

Fig. 3. Cost of gastric bypass versus savings in medication after gastric bypass. (*From* Snow LL, Weinstein LS, Hannon JK, et al. The effect of Roux-en-Y gastric bypass on prescription drug costs. Obes Surg 2005;14:1031–5; with permission.)

Bariatric surgery coverage by insurance companies

In North America, healthcare funding allocation has historically not been based on CEA or CBA but rather has been based on treatment effectiveness, with most effective treatments being covered regardless of their cost. Garber [54] reports that of 228 managed care plans surveyed nationwide, 93% cover a more effective yet more expensive intervention, with only 16% covering a new intervention if it is more expensive but no more effective. Only 40% of plans involved formal CEA for their policy making. The 1991 National Institutes of Health Consensus Development Panel stated that severe obesity (BMI $\geq$ 40 or slightly more than 100 pounds overweight) in and of itself met the criteria for weight loss surgery. Ironically, the effectiveness and cost effectiveness of surgical treatment of obesity and its serious comorbidities have been largely ignored by insurance companies.

The increasing demand for bariatric surgery has increased demands on private and public insurers to cover these effective procedures. To meet consumer demands, insurers are pressured to raise premiums, reduce reimbursement, increase copayments, or deny coverage. Frequently, physicians have difficulty with reimbursement for bariatric surgery procedures from insurers. Obesity is often viewed as an elective, cosmetic option, like plastic surgery rather, than a disease affecting all aspects of health and well-being. In these cases, patients are required to self-pay, often taking out loans. Most private insurance carriers add qualifiers to the guidelines laid down by the 1991 NIH Consensus Development Panel, such as a need for 6 or 12 months of a continuously medically supervised diet to qualify for reimbursement. Although most patients seeking weight loss surgery have accumulated years of failed diet treatments, these attempts are rarely associated with written documentation of those efforts.

Other insurance carriers deny coverage in their fine print. In Nebraska and Florida, the largest carrier, Blue Cross Blue Shield, discontinued health coverage for obesity surgery due to high demand and high costs [55]. Similarly, private insurers, such as Wal-Mart Corporation, CIGNA HealthCare, and Aetna Inc., deny coverage of bariatric surgery under their standard insurance plans [15]. In Arkansas, bariatric coverage was eliminated from its self-funded employee benefit plan as the morbidly obese population increased from 5% to 25% [56]. In the United States, federally governed Medicare or state-governed Medicaid insurance base their reimbursement on procedure codes recognized by an International Classification of Diseases (ICD) established by the WHO in ICD-9 and the most recent version of ICD-10 [26]. In ICD-9CM and ICD-10, endogenous obesity has a separate ICD code from that secondary to genetic or endocrine problems and therefore is not covered by Medicare or Medicaid. It was not until October 1, 2004 that the Centers for Medicare and Medicaid Services removed language from the National Coverage Determination Manual that "obesity itself cannot be considered an illness." This was a considerable step forward because it allowed consideration of obesity interventions that are supported by scientific and medical evidence. This did not result in obesity by itself warranting coverage of any bariatric surgical treatments. Another leap came in November of 2005 when the Centers for Medicare and Medicaid Services announced that the obesity policy will be modified to read as follows:

> Obesity may be caused by medical conditions such as hypothyroidism, Cushing's disease, and hypothalamic lesions or can aggravate a number of cardiac and respiratory diseases as well as diabetes and hypertension. Certain designated surgical services for the treatment of obesity are covered for Medicare beneficiaries who have a BMI ≥ 35, have at least one co-morbidity related to obesity and have been previously unsuccessful with the medical treatment of obesity. Treatments for obesity alone remain non-covered.

This change has resulted in better national coverage for bariatric surgery in the United States. Procedures that are often reimbursed include open and laparoscopic RYGB and laparoscopic AGB. Less frequently, insurance covers open and laparoscopic biliopancreatic diversion with duodenal switch. In general, all patients need to have at least one obesity-related health problem and have been previously unsuccessful with medical treatment for their obesity for their surgical procedure to be reimbursed.

In contrast to the United States, health plans in Canada pay for gastric bypass procedures. Gastric bypass is a general term that encompasses a variety of methods, all of which involve a reconfiguration of the digestive system. For example, in Ontario, the Ontario Health Insurance Plan Schedule of Benefits for Physician Services includes fee code "S120 gastric bypass or partition, for morbid obesity" as an insured service. Laparoscopic AGB is not covered by Ontario Health Insurance Plan or other Canadian plans.

Existing guidelines for the use of bariatric surgery

Societies, licensing boards, and governmental agencies have published guidelines to standardize care and encourage hospital investment in its infrastructure for their overweight patients. In 2003, high-volume hospitals (≥ 387 bariatric surgeries per year) had three times lower in-hospital deaths than low-volume hospitals (< 118 surgeries per year) [43]. The Betsy Lehman Center for Patient Safety and Medical Error Reduction convened an expert panel in Massachusetts to establish best practices for weight loss surgery (www.mass.gov/dph/betsylehman/panel_summary.htm) [57]. The American College of Surgeons has established the Bariatric Network to accredit hospitals based on Betsy Lehman guidelines and benchmarked outcomes. Similarly, the American Society for Bariatric Surgery has established an accreditation of surgeons and facilities based on volume, personnel, and infrastructure. In 2006, Blue Cross Blue Shield announced its intent to tie payment for bariatric surgery to Betsy Lehman guidelines, and the media has begun to profile hospitals that fall short of volume recommendations for

Centers of Excellence. In the most recent report from the November 2006 Blue Cross and Blue Shield Association Medical Advisory Panel meeting, laparoscopic AGB for morbid obesity was announced to meet the Technology Evaluation Center scientific criteria and is recommended for appropriately selected patients to be performed by trained surgeons in institutions that support a comprehensive bariatric surgery program, including long-term monitoring and follow-up post-surgery.

Summary

Obesity has reached epidemic proportions. Diet and exercise is rarely successful at sustained weight loss. In contrast, bariatric surgery achieves durable weight loss and often resolves costly comorbid illnesses, such as diabetes and hypertension. Laparoscopically performed weight loss procedures have emerged as cost-effective and efficacious alternatives to open bariatric surgery, offering decreased morbidity and mortality in selected patients. The societal expense of treating obesity is staggering, and national efforts must focus on obesity prevention. Once a patient is obese, denying access to surgical therapy is discriminatory, unjust, and does not make economic sense.

References

[1] Obesity in America. Obesity by the numbers. Available at: http://www.obesityinamerica.org/economicimpact.html. Accessed November 1, 2006.
[2] Martin LF, Robinson A, Moore BJ. Socioeconomic issues affecting the treatment of obesity in the new millennium. Pharmacoeconomics 2000;18:335–53.
[3] Tsai AG, Wadden TA, Womble LG, et al. Commercial and self-help programs for weight control. Psychiatr Clin North Am 2005;28:171–92.
[4] Manson JE, Willett WC, Stampfer MJ, et al. Body weight and mortality among women. N Engl J Med 1995;333:677–85.
[5] Fontaine KR, Redden DT, Wang C, et al. Years of life lost due to obesity. JAMA 2003;289:187–93.
[6] Flum DR, Dellinger EP. Impact of gastric bypass operation on survival: a population-based analysis. J Am Coll Surg 2004;199:543–51.
[7] Christou NV, Sampalis JS, Liberman M, et al. Surgery decreases long-term mortality, morbidity, and health care use in morbidly obese patients. Ann Surg 2004;240:416–23.
[8] World Health Organization. Controlling the global obesity epidemic. World Health Organization. Available at: http://www.who.int/nutrition/topics/obesity/en/. Accessed November 1, 2006.
[9] National Health and Nutrition Examination Survey (NHANES) report. Prevalence of overweight and obesity among adults: United States, 2003–2004. National Health and Nutrition Examination Survey (NHANES). Available at: http://www.cdc.gov/nchs/nhanes.htm. Accessed November 1, 2006.
[10] Ogden CL, Carroll MD, Curtin LR, et al. Prevalence of overweight and obesity in the United States, 1999–2004. JAMA 2006;295:1549–55.
[11] Magarey AM, Daniels LA, Boulton TJ, et al. Predicting obesity in early adulthood from childhood and parental obesity. Int J Obes Relat Metab Disord 2003;27:505–13.

[12] Statistics Canada. Canadian Community Health Survey. Statistics Canada. Available at: http://www.statcan.ca/english/research/82-620-MIE/2005001/tables.htm. Accessed November 1, 2006.

[13] World Health Organization. Obesity: preventing and managing the global epidemic. Technical Report Series no.894. Geneva (Switzerland):WHO; 2000.

[14] National Institutes of Health. National Institute of Diabetes, Digestive and Kidney Diseases. Statistics related to overweight and obesity: the economic costs. Available at: http://www.win.niddk.nih.gov/statistics/index.htm. Accessed November 1, 2006.

[15] Finkelstein EA, Fiebelkorn IC, Wang G. National medical spending attributable to overweight and obesity: how much, and who's paying? Health Aff (Millwood) 2003;W3(Suppl Web Exclusives):219–26.

[16] Finkelstein EA, Fiebelkorn IC, Wang G. State-level estimates of annual medical expenditures attributable to obesity. Obes Res 2004;12:18–24.

[17] National Cancer Institute. Cancer trends progress report 2005 update. National Cancer Institute. Available at: http://progressreport.cancer.gov/doc_detail.asp?pid=1&did=2005&chid=25&coid=226&mid=. Accessed November 2, 2006.

[18] Martin LF, Lundberg AP, Juneau F, et al. A description of morbidly obese state employees requesting a bariatric operation. Surgery 2005;138:690–700.

[19] Daviglus ML, Liu K, Yan LL, et al. Relation of body mass index in young adulthood and middle age to Medicare expenditures in older age. JAMA 2004;292:2743–9.

[20] Birmingham CL, Muller JL, Palepu A, et al. The cost of obesity in Canada. CMAJ 1999;160:483–8.

[21] Katzmarzyk PT, Janssen I. The economic costs associated with physical inactivity and obesity in Canada: an update. Can J Appl Physiol 2004;29:90–115.

[22] Sturm R. The effects of obesity, smoking, and drinking on medical problems and costs. Health Aff (Millwood) 2002;21:245–53.

[23] Thompson D, Edelsberg J, Kinsey KL, et al. Estimated economic costs of obesity to U.S. business. Am J Health Promot 1998;13:120–7.

[24] Finkelstein E, Fiebelkorn C, Wang G. The costs of obesity among full-time employees. Am J Health Promot 2005;20:45–51.

[25] Frezza EE, Wachtel MS, Ewing BT. The impact of morbid obesity on the state economy: an initial evaluation. Surg Obes Relat Dis 2006;2:504–8.

[26] Martin LF, White S, Lindstrom W Jr. Cost-benefit analysis for the treatment of severe obesity. World J Surg 1998;22:1008–17.

[27] Swinburn BA, Caterson I, Seidell JC, et al. Diet, nutrition and the prevention of excess weight gain and obesity. Public Health Nutr 2004;7:123–46.

[28] Chou SY, Grossman M, Saffer H. An economic analysis of adult obesity: results from the behavioral risk factor surveillance system. J Health Econ 2004;23:565–87.

[29] Philipson TJ, Posner RA. The long-run growth in obesity as a function of technological change. Perspect Biol Med 2003;46:S87–107.

[30] Norris SL, Zhang X, Avenell A, et al. Pharmacotherapy for weight loss in adults with type 2 diabetes mellitus. Cochrane Database Syst Rev 2005;CD004096.

[31] Gastrointestinal surgery for severe obesity. Proceedings of a National Institutes of Health Consensus Development Conference. March 25–27, 1991, Bethesda, MD. Am J Clin Nutr 1992;55:487S–619S.

[32] Medical Advisory Secretariat. Ontario Ministry of Health and Long-Term Care Government of Ontario. Bariatric Surgery Health Technology Literature Review 2005.

[33] Buchwald H, Avidor Y, Braunwald E, et al. Bariatric surgery: a systematic review and meta-analysis. JAMA 2004;292:1724–37.

[34] American Diabetes Association. Direct and indirect costs of diabetes in the United States. American Diabetes Association. Available at: www.diabetes.org. Accessed November 1, 2006.

[35] Sjostrom L, Lindroos AK, Peltonen M, et al. Lifestyle, diabetes, and cardiovascular risk factors 10 years after bariatric surgery. N Engl J Med 2004;351:2683–93.

[36] Puzziferri N, Austrheim-Smith IT, Wolfe BM, et al. Three-year follow-up of a prospective randomized trial comparing laparoscopic versus open gastric bypass. Ann Surg 2006;243: 181–8.

[37] Clegg A, Colquitt J, Sidhu M, et al. Clinical and cost effectiveness of surgery for morbid obesity: a systematic review and economic evaluation. Int J Obes Relat Metab Disord 2003;27: 1167–77.

[38] Siddiqui A, Livingston E, Huerta S. A comparison of open and laparoscopic Roux-en-Y gastric bypass surgery for morbid and super obesity: a decision-analysis model. Am J Surg 2006; 192:e1–7.

[39] Smith SC, Edwards CB, Goodman GN, et al. Open vs laparoscopic Roux-en-Y gastric bypass: comparison of operative morbidity and mortality. Obes Surg 2004;14:73–6.

[40] Santry HP, Gillen DL, Lauderdale DS. Trends in bariatric surgical procedures. JAMA 2005; 294:1909–17.

[41] Encinosa WE, Bernard DM, Steiner CA, et al. Use and costs of bariatric surgery and prescription weight-loss medications. Health Aff (Millwood) 2005;24:1039–46.

[42] Scopinaro N. The IFSO and obesity surgery throughout the world. International Federation for the Surgery of Obesity. Obes Surg 1998;8:3–8.

[43] HCUP NIS Database Documentation. Healthcare cost and utilization project (HCUP). Agency for Healthcare Research and Quality, Rockville (MD). Available at: http://www. ahrq.gov/research/may06/0506RA20.htm. Accessed November 1, 2006.

[44] Paxton JH, Matthews JB. The cost effectiveness of laparoscopic versus open gastric bypass surgery. Obes Surg 2005;15:24–34.

[45] Livingston EH. Hospital costs associated with bariatric procedures in the United States. Am J Surg 2005;190:816–20.

[46] Salem L, Jensen CC, Flum DR. Are bariatric surgical outcomes worth their cost? A systematic review. J Am Coll Surg 2005;200:270–8.

[47] van Gemert WG, Adang EM, Kop M, et al. A prospective cost-effectiveness analysis of vertical banded gastroplasty for the treatment of morbid obesity. Obes Surg 1999;9:484–91.

[48] Craig BM, Tseng DS. Cost-effectiveness of gastric bypass for severe obesity. Am J Med 2002; 113:491–8.

[49] Sampalis JS, Liberman M, Auger S, et al. The impact of weight reduction surgery on healthcare costs in morbidly obese patients. Obes Surg 2004;14:939–47.

[50] Solomon CG, Dluhy RG. Bariatric surgery: quick fix or long-term solution? N Engl J Med 2004;351:2751–3.

[51] Monk JS Jr, Dia NN, Stehr W. Pharmaceutical savings after gastric bypass surgery. Obes Surg 2004;14:13–5.

[52] Snow LL, Weinstein LS, Hannon JK, et al. The effect of Roux-en-Y gastric bypass on prescription drug costs. Obes Surg 2004;14:1031–5.

[53] Narbro K, Agren G, Jonsson E, et al. Pharmaceutical costs in obese individuals: comparison with a randomly selected population sample and long-term changes after conventional and surgical treatment: the SOS intervention study. Arch Intern Med 2002;162:2061–9.

[54] Garber AM. Cost-effectiveness and evidence evaluation as criteria for coverage policy. Health Aff (Millwood) 2004;W4(Suppl Web Exclusives):96.

[55] Stein R. As obesity surgeries soar, so do safety, cost concerns. Washington Post. November 5, 2006;A01.

[56] Alt SJ. Bariatric surgery may become a self-pay service. Health Care Strateg Manage 2003; 21(12):1,12–9.

[57] Kelly J, Tarnoff M, Shikora S, et al. Best practice recommendations for surgical care in weight loss surgery. Obes Res. 2005;13:227–33.

ELSEVIER
SAUNDERS

THE MEDICAL
CLINICS
OF NORTH AMERICA

Med Clin N Am 91 (2007) 339–351

Preoperative Assessment and Perioperative Care of Patients Undergoing Bariatric Surgery

Rajesh Kuruba, MD[a,b], Lisa S. Koche, MD[b,c],
Michel M. Murr, MD, FACS[a,b],*

[a]*Department of Bariatric Surgery, University of South Florida, c/o Tampa General Hospital,
P.O. Box 1289, Suite F-145, Tampa, FL 33601, USA*
[b]*Weight Management and Metabolic Health Center, P.O. Box 1289, Suite F-145,
Tampa, FL 33601, USA*
[c]*Spectra Complete Healthcare, University of South Florida, 509 South Armenia Avenue,
Suite #302, Tampa, FL 33609, USA*

The prevalence of morbid obesity in the United States and worldwide is increasing at an alarming rate. Between 1986 and 2000, the prevalence of adult Americans who have a body mass index (BMI) 40 kg/m^2 or greater quadrupled [1]. The recent National Health and Nutrition Examination Survey for 1999 through 2000 showed significant increases in the prevalence obesity (BMI ≥ 30 kg/m^2) from 23% to 31% and increases in extreme or morbid obesity (BMI ≥ 40 kg/m^2) from 2.9% to 4.7% compared with 1988 through 1994 [2]. The number of bariatric surgical procedures also has steadily increased during the past decade from 13,365 procedures in 1998 to 71,177 procedures in 2002 [3] and was expected to reach 140,000 in 2004 as a result of the increasing prevalence of morbid obesity, inconsistent weight loss with nonoperative therapy, and increasing evidence that bariatric procedures result in significant and durable weight loss, improve comorbid conditions, and reduce health care expenditure.

Although the overall mortality and morbidity rates of bariatric surgery are less than 1% and 15%, respectively [4,5], certain groups are at higher risk for complications [4,6] because of the high burden of comorbidities. There are three central questions to the suitability of patients for bariatric surgery: (1) Are patients ready and well equipped for lifelong changes?

---

* Corresponding author. Department of Bariatric Surgery, University of South Florida, c/o Tampa General Hospital, P.O. Box 1289 Suite F-145, Tampa, FL 33601.
E-mail address: mmurr@health.usf.edu (M.M. Murr).

0025-7125/07/$ - see front matter © 2007 Published by Elsevier Inc.
doi:10.1016/j.mcna.2007.01.010   *medical.theclinics.com*

(2) What are the optimal methods to assess their operative risk? and (3) What is the best model for interdisciplinary care that these patients need? This article reviews the published literature and current practice trends for preoperative workup and assessment of patients undergoing bariatric surgery.

Preoperative assessment

Candidates for bariatric procedures should be selected carefully after evaluation by an interdisciplinary team with access to medical, surgical, psychiatric, and nutritional expertise (Fig. 1). The goals of preoperative assessment for bariatric surgery are listed in Box 1, and criteria for bariatric surgery are listed in Box 2.

Contraindications for bariatric procedures

There are a few absolute contraindications to bariatric surgery, such as mental/cognitive impairment, active cancer, advanced liver disease with

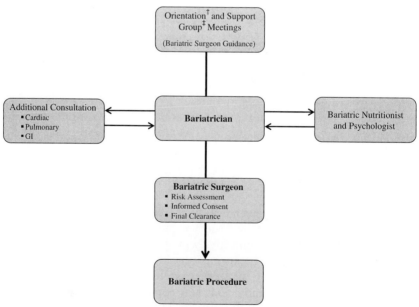

†Orientation meeting: Overview of the requirements (including third party payers) and process of weight loss surgery program.

‡Support group meeting: Candidates for bariatric surgery have the opportunity to talk to postoperative bariatric patients who can provide information relevant to pre- and postoperative issues.

Fig. 1. Our algorithm for evaluation and preoperative assessment of bariatric patients.

Box 1. Goals of preoperative assessment for bariatric surgery

Assess indications and contraindications to operative treatment.
Perform comprehensive and interdisciplinary medical,
psychological, and dietary evaluations.
Treat and optimize medical comorbidities before surgical
intervention.
Educate the patients and their support system about options of
treatment and risk and set realistic expectations.

---

portal hypertension, unstable coronary artery disease, and uncontrolled severe obstructive sleep apnea with pulmonary hypertension (pulmonary systolic pressure > 50 mm Hg). Age is no longer considered an absolute contraindication to bariatric surgery [9,10].

Role of the bariatric surgeon

The bariatric surgeon should be the key person to coordinate an interdisciplinary team and supervise preoperative evaluation along with a bariatrician. A decision for bariatric surgery should be reached, preferably along with family members, only after assessment of the probability that the patient will be able to tolerate surgery without excessive risk and will comply with the postoperative regimen and life-long medical surveillance.

Role of the bariatric nutritionist

The purpose of dietary counseling is not to induce weight loss preoperatively but to assess the patient's nutritional status and aid in patient education. Registered dietitians are best qualified to provide nutritional care, including preoperative assessment and postoperative education, counseling, follow-up [11,12], and education to patients about self-monitoring, meal planning, assessing nutritional deficiencies, and nutritional

---

Box 2. Criteria for bariatric surgery

As per the NIH consensus conference, eligibility for bariatric
surgery is summarized as follows [7,8]:
BMI ≥ 40 kg/m^2 or ≥ 35 kg/m^2 with comorbid conditions
Failure of nonoperative weight loss efforts
Absence of contraindications (medical and psychological)
Well informed, compliant, and motivated patient

---

supplementation. Postoperatively, patients are required to take life-long nutritional supplements and to undergo life-long medical monitoring. Dedicated dietitians with specialty training in nutritional medicine are instrumental in the preoperative education of patients on new dietary requirements and stipulations and adjustment to those requirements after weight loss surgery.

Role of the bariatric psychologist/psychiatrist

Bariatric patients have a high prevalence of depression, anxiety, binge eating, night eating syndrome, post-traumatic stress disorder, and body dysmorphic disorders; approximately half of bariatric patients are taking psychotropic medications [13]. A preoperative evaluation should aim to assess a patient's psychological well-being, ability to make informed decisions, and willingness to participate actively in postoperative treatment [14]. In a systematic review of 29 studies, serious psychiatric disorders that required inpatient hospitalization and personality disorders were found to predict suboptimal weight loss after surgery [15].

Although there is no standardized protocol for the psychiatric and psychological evaluation of patients undergoing bariatric surgery, many centers use a structured interview, such as the Boston interview for gastric bypass [14], guidelines from Montefiore Medial Center/Albert Einstein College of Medicine [16], and the Weight and Lifestyle Inventory from the University of Pennsylvania [17]. Additionally, many clinicians use the Beck Depression Inventory or the Minnesota Multiphasic Personality Inventory for psychological testing [18].

We use brief motivational interviewing to assess the patients' readiness for change and to set realistic expectations of weight loss. In a survey of 230 women and 54 men, we found that patients' "dream weight" was 89% ± 8% excess body weight loss and that 67% ± 10% and 49% ± 14% excess body weight loss are "acceptable" and "disappointing" weights, respectively. These unrealistic weight loss expectations should be addressed to avoid regressive behavior postoperatively [19].

Role of the bariatrician

An internist or primary care provider with strong interest and training in bariatrics should ensure proper preoperative evaluation and treatment of comorbidities before and after bariatric surgery. A detailed history of nutrition, weight loss or gain, and physical activity should be obtained, and secondary causes of obesity (eg, Cushing syndrome, hypothyroidism) should be assessed and ruled out when clinically suspected. Although routine laboratory studies in the absence of physical findings are controversial [20], a list of commonly recommended tests is detailed in Table 1. Additional diagnostic

Table 1
Recommended preoperative testing

Test	Indication
Complete blood count	
Comprehensive metabolic panel, liver function tests	Renal failure, congestive heart failure, diuretic use, NASH
Creatinine	Age >50 yr, diuretic use
PT/PTT	Malnutrition (revisional bariatric surgery)
Glucose, Hb A1c	Obesity or DM
Electrocardiogram	Men >40 yr, women >50 yr, known coronary artery disease, hypertension, diabetes
Chest radiograph	Age >50 yr, known or suspected cardiac or pulmonary disease

Abbreviations: DM, diabetes mellitus; NASH, nonalcoholic steatosis; PT/PTT, prothrombin time/partial thromboplastin time.

testing and expert consultations (eg, with cardiologists, pulmonologists, and gastroenterologists) should be obtained when clinically indicated. Another goal of preoperative evaluation is to provide patients with guidelines and goals to increase their physical activity. Specifically, the bariatrician should assess preoperative patients as follows.

Endocrine

Strict glycemic control during the perioperative period to maintain serum glucose below 150 mg/dL or HBA1C <7 is essential to reduce adverse events. Routine screening for secondary causes of obesity, such as Cushing syndrome or hypothyroidism, has not been proven to be beneficial because of the rarity of these disorders compared with the epidemic of exogenous obesity in this context.

Cardiac

Patients should be assessed for cardiac risk according to the American Heart Association guidelines [21]. Patients should be assessed for risk based on history and physical and functional capacity. Intermediate- or high-risk patients require further cardiac evaluation; a reliable clinical predictor is the patient's ability to perform activities requiring at least four metabolic equivalents (eg, climbing a flight of stairs or walking up a hill).

Full evaluation may not be feasible because of body habitus and weight limitations of diagnostic equipment. The accuracy of thallium-201 scanning can be significantly diminished in patients who have a BMI greater than 30 kg/m^2 [22]. Transesophageal dobutamine stress echocardiography may be superior to the other types of stress echocardiography testing for obese patients [23]. Beta-blockers may decrease the risk of perioperative ischemia, infarction, or dysrhythmia in patients who have coronary artery disease [21], but its role is not defined in bariatric surgery.

We screen asymptomatic patients for coronary disease if they have at least one of the following: age greater than 50 years with at least two of the following: metabolic syndrome, diabetes, hypertension, smoking, dyslipidemia, or family history of coronary disease; an abnormal baseline electrocardiogram; or prior history of coronary artery disease/valvular disease.

Using this protocol, we screen 25% to 35% of patients who are asymptomatic and 10% of patients who have known coronary artery disease. Nuclear imaging detects abnormalities in 5% of the told cohort that require further intervention. We treat high-risk patients or patients who have coronary artery disease with perioperative beta-blockers starting 1 week preoperatively and up to 2 weeks postoperatively.

Pulmonary

Obstructive sleep apnea (OSA) is characterized by periodic, partial, or complete obstruction of the upper airway during sleep. The prevalence of OSA in large series of bariatric surgical patients is 39% to 71% [24,25]. The American Society of Anesthesiologists practice parameters are useful for the perioperative assessment and management of patients who have OSA [26]. Preoperative initiation and perioperative use of continuous positive airway pressure (CPAP) or bilevel positive airway pressure (BiPAP) can reduce hypercarbia, hypoxemia, and pulmonary artery vasoconstriction.

We screen patients by history, neck examination, and the Epworth Sleepiness Scale (Table 2) and refer them to polysomnography if they score 6 or higher on the Epworth Sleepiness Scale and if they snore [27,28]. Using these criteria, we refer 75% of all bariatric patients for polysomnography, the majority of whom (82%) are diagnosed with OSA. We require at least 4 weeks of treatment with CPAP/BiPAP before the proposed operation to minimize

Table 2
Epworth sleepiness scale

Situation	Chance of dozing[a]
Sitting and reading	
Watching TV	
Sitting, inactive in a public place (eg, a theater or a meeting)	
As a passenger in a car for an hour without a break	
Lying down to rest in the afternoon when circumstances permit	
Sitting and talking to someone	
Sitting quietly after a lunch without alcohol	
Ina car, while stopped for a few minutes in the traffic	
Total	
Do you snore while sleeping?	☐Yes—☐No
Does your bed partner say that you snore?	☐Yes—☐No

[a] 0 = none; 1 = slight; 2 = moderate; 3 = high.

alveolar hypoventilation. Additionally, we reinstitute CPAP/BiPAP treatment in the recovery room and during day- and night-time sleep in the immediate postoperative period. With this approach, the incidence of postoperative primary respiratory failure in our cohort is 1% [29]. Occasionally, we require pulmonary function tests and spirometry in patients who have known reactive airways disease and chronic obstructive pulmonary disease.

Hypercoagulability

Obesity is an independent risk factor for venothromboembolic events (VTE). This risk is accentuated by pneumoperitoneum during surgery and perioperative hypercoagulability through increased levels of fibrinogen, factor VIII, and von Willebrand factor. The incidence of VTE in patients receiving routine perioperative prophylaxis ranges from 0.2% to 3.5% [30,31]. Although 95% of bariatric surgeons use some form of thromboprophylaxis routinely [32], clear dosing guidelines for prophylaxis of VTE in bariatric patients have not been developed because of the elusive relationship of body weight and dosing regimens and because many of the studies that compared different regimens and doses were underpowered [33,34]. However, VTE prophylaxis and early ambulation should be pursued in all patients.

The role of routine duplex ultrasonography in detecting deep venous thrombosis is not clear and cannot be justified in bariatric patients. Prophylactic inferior vena cava filter placement may be beneficial for bariatric patients at high risk for postoperative VTE (eg, patients who have venous stasis disease, BMI ≥ 60 kg/m^2, truncal obesity, prior VTE, and known hypercoagulable state) [31,35,36]. Extended prophylaxis (postdischarge) with low-molecular-weight heparin may be necessary for these high-risk patients.

We use 7500 units of unfractionated heparin subcutaneously on call to the operating room and use enoxaparin 40 mg subcutaneously daily for patients who have a BMI 50 kg/m^2 or greater and 30 mg subcutaneously twice daily for patients who have a BMI greater than 50 kg/m^2 until discharged from the hospital. We use extended prophylaxis with enoxaparin 60 mg subcutaneously daily for 10 days after discharge from the hospital for patients who have a BMI 60 kg/m^2 or greater, relative immobility, or previous history of VTE.

Gastrointestinal

The recent European guideline that strongly recommends upper endoscopy or contrast studies before gastric bypass [37] is based on a single study that showed significant upper gastrointestinal tract lesions in 62% of patients [38]. Potential drawbacks for screening asymptomatic patients include low impact of endoscopy on surgical management and the secondary unnecessary work-up prompted by endoscopic findings and its attendant increased costs [39–41]. The recommendations to screen for *Helicobacter pylori* in asymptomatic bariatric patients are not well founded.

Obesity is a risk factor for cholelithiasis. Gallstone formation is common after bariatric surgery due to rapid weight loss and occurs in 32% of patients within 6 months of gastric bypass [42]. For these reasons and because of the impracticality of screening all patients preoperatively, we undertake a routine cholecystectomy at the time of gastric bypass [43]. Other clinicians prefer a selective approach and remove only gallbladders that contain stones; if cholecystectomy is not performed at the time of surgery, ursodiol 600 mg daily for 6 months may reduce the incidence of new stone formation [42].

In summary, we do not routinely screen for gallstones, hiatal hernias, or *H pylori* in asymptomatic patients.

Liver

Nonalcoholic fatty liver disease (NAFLD) is a clinicopathologic condition characterized by significant lipid deposition in hepatocytes that may induce a wide spectrum of liver damage ranging from simple fatty infiltration to cirrhosis. When inflammatory changes occur with or without fibrosis, the term "nonalcoholic steatohepatitis" (NASH) is more appropriate.

In a review of 12 observational studies including 1620 patients, the prevalence of steatosis was 91% (range, 85%–98%), the prevalence of NASH was 37% (range, 24%–98%), and the prevalence of unexpected cirrhosis was 1.7% (range, 1%–7%) [44]. Patients older than 45 years and those who were obese or diabetic are at greatest risk for advanced fibrosis [45,46].

Preoperative assessment for bariatric patients should include comprehensive liver function panel, lipid profile, and, when indicated, viral markers for hepatitis. Because clinical and radiologic parameters of the presence or severity of NAFLD/NASH are unreliable and preoperative liver biopsies are impractical, we routinely obtain a liver biopsy during the bariatric surgical procedure to diagnose and stage NAFLD/NASH [47,48]. Earlier bariatric surgical procedures, such as the jejunoileal bypass [49], with too rapid a weight loss along with the attendant malnutrition had adverse effect on liver function. Contemporary surgical procedures, such as gastric bypass with more controlled weight loss, have shown to improve NASH, including fibrosis [50,51]. Patients who have known cirrhosis and impairment of hepatic reserve (eg, Childs-Pugh class B or C) or the presence of portal hypertension or ascites are at prohibitive risk for complications.

Recommendations for preoperative diets that reduce liver size are not founded in rigorous scientific data and warrant further studies.

Dysfertility

At least 50% of patients who have polycystic ovary syndrome (PCOS) are obese [52]. PCOS is diagnosed by the presence of at least two of the following criteria: oligo- or anovulation, clinical or biochemical signs of hyperandrogenism, and polycystic ovaries [53].

The endocrine abnormalities of PCOS include increased serum androgens, increased luteinizing hormone level, increased luteinizing hormone/follicle-stimulating hormone ratio, and hyperinsulinemia. Weight loss and very-low-calorie diets lead to normalization of insulin resistance, menstrual dysfunction, and oligo-ovulation. Because diet-based and pharmacologic therapies do not lead to sustained weight loss, interest in bariatric surgery for amelioration of PCOS has risen. In a series of 24 patients who had PCOS and mean BMI of 50 ± 8 kg/m^2, gastric bypass resulted in significant improvement of manifestations related to PCOS [54].

Preoperative risk scoring

The overall mortality of bariatric surgery is less than 1% [4,55]. Recently, higher mortality rates have been reported among Medicare beneficiaries and patients older than 65 years of age [6]. Male gender, older age, high BMI, and surgeon's experience have been identified as predictors of adverse events by multivariate analysis [4,6,56]. The Obesity Surgery Mortality Risk Score, which was developed by DeMaria and colleagues (Eric DeMaria, MD, FACS, personal communication, 2006), uses five patient characteristics. Age 45 years or greater, hypertension, BMI 50 kg/m^2 or greater, male gender, and risk of pulmonary embolism (history of VTE, pulmonary hypertension, and obesity hypoventilation) have been proposed to predict perioperative mortality of bariatric surgery. In a multicenter study of 4433 patients, including our cohort, to validate the OSMRS, patients who had 0 to 1, 2 to 3, or 4 to 5 risk factors had mortality rates of 0.37%, 1.21% and 2.4%, respectively. This risk stratification may help in surgical decision making and in obtaining informed consent and may allow standardization of outcome comparisons between different centers.

Anesthetic considerations

Preoperative evaluation

Attention should focus on issues unique to the obese patient, particularly cardiorespiratory status and the airway. With severe pulmonary hypertension, pulmonary artery catheterization and monitoring may be necessary. Preoperative arterial blood gas can identify carbon dioxide retention, provide guidelines for perioperative oxygen requirements, and aid in setting guidelines for weaning from the ventilator during the postoperative period.

It is recommended that the patient's usual medications, except insulin, diuretics, and oral hypoglycemics, be continued until the time of surgery. Antibiotic prophylaxis is important because of the increased risk of postoperative wound infection.

Intraoperative care

Operating room beds with a high weight capacity are required. The patient should be well secured because of the risk for falling during table position changes. Particular care should be paid to protect pressure areas during positioning because pressure sores and neural injuries are more common in obese patients.

Endotracheal intubation and airway management in the obese patient can be challenging, and a number of clinical factors can predict ventilation and tracheal intubation difficulty: primarily neck circumference [57], visualization of oropharyngeal structures (Mallampati score), thyromental distance, and dental configuration. Brodsky and colleagues [57], in a study of 100 morbidly obese patients, found that neither obesity nor BMI predicted difficult intubation, whereas a high Mallampati score (≥ 3) and large neck circumference increased the potential for difficult laryngoscopy and intubation. Towels or a shoulder roll can be used to extend the neck. Optimal positioning of the patient and consideration of an algorithm for difficult airway management, such as the American Society of Anesthesiologists' Practice Guidelines for Management of the Difficult Airway, help to achieve safe and rapid airway management [26].

Blood pressure cuffs should span a minimum of 75% of the patient's upper arm circumference for reliable measurements. Invasive arterial monitoring should be used for the "super" obese (BMI ≥ 60 kg/m^2), for patients who have severe cardiopulmonary disease, or for patients in whom the noninvasive blood pressure cuff reading is unreliable. Central venous catheters should be used in cases of difficult peripheral venous access or when postoperative access may be difficult. Highly lipophilic substances, such as barbiturates and benzodiazepines [58], show significant increases in the volume of distribution for obese individuals relative to normal-weight individuals, and these drugs must be administered in higher doses. Desflurane has been suggested as the inhaled anesthetic of choice in this patient population because of its more rapid and consistent recovery profile. Complete muscular relaxation is crucial during laparoscopic bariatric procedures to facilitate ventilation and to maintain an adequate working space for visualization and safe manipulation of laparoscopic instruments. Collapse of the pneumoperitoneum may be an early indication that muscle relaxation is inadequate.

Postoperative considerations

Patients who have significant cardiac disease, male gender, BMI 60 kg/m^2 or greater, diabetes, OSA, and intraoperative complications are the risk factors predictive of postoperative ICU admission [59]. We manage all of our patients in a specialized nursing unit for bariatric patients; routine admissions to the ICU are < 1%. Patients who need intravenous beta-blockers are monitored by telemetry.

Summary

The field of bariatric surgery has changed dramatically since the NIH Consensus Conference statement in 1991. As bariatric surgeons continue to improve procedures for weight loss, successful outcomes after bariatric surgery depend not only on the technical expertise of the surgeon but also on careful preoperative assessment, screening, and minimization of preoperative risk. Further research is needed for formulating evidence based on the guidelines for many aspects of the perioperative care of bariatric patients.

References

[1] Sturm R. Increases in clinically severe obesity in the United States, 1986–2000. Arch Intern Med 2003;163:2146–8.

[2] Flegal KM, Carroll MD, Ogden CL, et al. Prevalence and trends in obesity among US adults, 1999–2000. JAMA 2002;288:1723–7.

[3] Santry HP, Gillen DL, Lauderdale DS. Trends in bariatric surgical procedures. JAMA 2005; 294:1909–17.

[4] Murr MM, Martin T, Haines KL, et al. A state wide review of contemporary outcomes of gastric bypass in Florida. Does provider volume impact outcomes? Ann Surg, in press.

[5] Podnos YD, Jimenez JC, Wilson SE, et al. Complications after laparoscopic gastric bypass: a review of 3464 cases. Arch Surg 2003;138:957–61.

[6] Flum DR, Salem L, Elrod JA, et al. Early mortality among Medicare beneficiaries undergoing bariatric surgical procedures. JAMA 2005;294:1903–8.

[7] National Institutes of Health Consensus Development Panel. Gastrointestinal surgery for severe obesity. Proceedings of a National Institutes of Health Consensus Development Conference (Publication #NIH 98-4083). March 25–27, 1991, Bethesda, MD. Am J Clin Nutr 1992;55:487S–619S.

[8] NHLBI Obesity Education Initiative Expert Panel on the Identification, Evaluation, and Treatment of Overweight and Obesity in Adults. Clinical guidelines on the identification, evaluation, and treatment of overweight and obesity in adults–the evidence report. National Institutes of Health. Obes Res 1998;6(Suppl 2):51S–209S.

[9] Nelson LG, Lopez PP, Haines K, et al. Outcomes of bariatric surgery in patients > or = 65 years. Surg Obes Relat Dis 2006;2:384–8.

[10] Murr MM, Siadati MR, Sarr MG. Results of bariatric surgery for morbid obesity in patients older than 50 years. Obes Surg 1995;5:399–402.

[11] Fobi MA. Surgical treatment of obesity: a review. J Natl Med Assoc 2004;96:61–75.

[12] Bond DS, Evans RK, DeMaria EJ, et al. A conceptual application of health behavior theory in the design and implementation of a successful surgical weight loss program. Obes Surg 2004;14:849–56.

[13] Pawlow LA, O'Neil PM, White MA, et al. Findings and outcomes of psychological evaluations of gastric bypass applicants. Surg Obes Relat Dis 2005;1:523–7 [discussion: 528–9].

[14] Sogg S, Mori DL. The Boston interview for gastric bypass: determining the psychological suitability of surgical candidates. Obes Surg 2004;14:370–80.

[15] Herpertz S, Kielmann R, Wolf AM, et al. Do psychosocial variables predict weight loss or mental health after obesity surgery? A systematic review. Obes Res 2004;12:1554–69.

[16] Glinski J, Wetzler S, Goodman E. The psychology of gastric bypass surgery. Obes Surg 2001; 11:581–8.

[17] Wadden TA, Sarwer DB. Behavioral assessment of candidates for bariatric surgery: a patient-oriented approach. Surg Obes Relat Dis 2006;2:171–9.

[18] Bauchowitz AU, Gonder-Frederick LA, Olbrisch ME, et al. Psychosocial evaluation of bariatric surgery candidates: a survey of present practices. Psychosom Med 2005;67:825–32.

[19] Kaly P, Orellana S, Takagishi C, et al. Unrealistic weight loss expectations in candidates for bariatric surgery. San Francisco (CA): American Society for Bariatric Surgery; 2006.

[20] Smetana GW, Macpherson DS. The case against routine preoperative laboratory testing. Med Clin North Am 2003;87:7–40.

[21] Eagle KA, Berger PB, Calkins H, et al. ACC/AHA guideline update for perioperative cardiovascular evaluation for noncardiac surgery–executive summary: a report of the American College of Cardiology/American Heart Association Task Force on Practice Guidelines (Committee to Update the 1996 Guidelines on Perioperative Cardiovascular Evaluation for Noncardiac Surgery). J Am Coll Cardiol 2002;39:542–53.

[22] Hansen CL, Woodhouse S, Kramer M. Effect of patient obesity on the accuracy of thallium-201 myocardial perfusion imaging. Am J Cardiol 2000;85:749–52.

[23] Vitarelli A, Dagianti A, Conde Y, et al. Value of transesophageal dobutamine stress echocardiography in assessing coronary artery disease. Am J Cardiol 2000;86:57G–60G.

[24] Byhahn C, Lischke V, Meininger D, et al. Peri-operative complications during percutaneous tracheostomy in obese patients. Anaesthesia 2005;60:12–5.

[25] Frey WC, Pilcher J. Obstructive sleep-related breathing disorders in patients evaluated for bariatric surgery. Obes Surg 2003;13:676–83.

[26] American Society of Anesthesiologists Task Force on Management of the Difficult Airway. Practice guidelines for management of the difficult airway: an updated report. Anesthesiology 2003;98:1269–77.

[27] Serafini FM, MacDowell Anderson W, Rosemurgy AS, et al. Clinical predictors of sleep apnea in patients undergoing bariatric surgery. Obes Surg 2001;11:28–31.

[28] Rasheid S, Banasiak M, Gallagher SF, et al. Gastric bypass is an effective treatment for obstructive sleep apnea in patients with clinically significant obesity. Obes Surg 2003;13:58–61.

[29] Haines K, Nelson LG, Gonzalez R, et al. Objective evidence that bariatric surgery improves obesity-related obstructive sleep apnea. Surgery, in press.

[30] Higa KD, Boone KB, Ho T. Complications of the laparoscopic Roux-en-Y gastric bypass: 1,040 patients–what have we learned? Obes Surg 2000;10:509–13.

[31] Gonzalez R, Haines K, Nelson LG, et al. Predictive factors of thromboembolic events in patients undergoing Roux-en-Y gastric bypass. Surg Obes Relat Dis 2006;2:30–5 [discussion: 35–6].

[32] Wu EC, Barba CA. Current practices in the prophylaxis of venous thromboembolism in bariatric surgery. Obes Surg 2000;10:7–13 [discussion: 14].

[33] Scholten DJ, Hoedema RM, Scholten SE. A comparison of two different prophylactic dose regimens of low molecular weight heparin in bariatric surgery. Obes Surg 2002;12:19–24.

[34] Miller MT, Rovito PF. An approach to venous thromboembolism prophylaxis in laparoscopic Roux-en-Y gastric bypass surgery. Obes Surg 2004;14:731–7.

[35] Sapala JA, Wood MH, Schuhknecht MP, et al. Fatal pulmonary embolism after bariatric operations for morbid obesity: a 24-year retrospective analysis. Obes Surg 2003;13:819–25.

[36] Keeling WB, Haines K, Stone PA, et al. Current indications for preoperative inferior vena cava filter insertion in patients undergoing surgery for morbid obesity. Obes Surg 2005;15:1009–12.

[37] Sauerland S, Angrisani L, Belachew M, et al. Obesity surgery: evidence-based guidelines of the European Association for Endoscopic Surgery (EAES). Surg Endosc 2005;19:200–21.

[38] Sharaf RN, Weinshel EH, Bini EJ, et al. Endoscopy plays an important preoperative role in bariatric surgery. Obes Surg 2004;14:1367–72.

[39] Madan AK, Speck KE, Hiler ML. Routine preoperative upper endoscopy for laparoscopic gastric bypass: is it necessary? Am Surg 2004;70:684–6.

[40] Ghassemian AJ, MacDonald KG, Cunningham PG, et al. The workup for bariatric surgery does not require a routine upper gastrointestinal series. Obes Surg 1997;7:16–8.

[41] Azagury D, Dumonceau JM, Morel P, et al. Preoperative work-up in asymptomatic patients undergoing Roux-en-Y gastric bypass: is endoscopy mandatory? Obes Surg 2006;16: 1304–11.
[42] Sugerman HJ, Brewer WH, Shiffman ML, et al. A multicenter, placebo-controlled, randomized, double-blind, prospective trial of prophylactic ursodiol for the prevention of gallstone formation following gastric-bypass-induced rapid weight loss. Am J Surg 1995;169:91–6 [discussion: 96–7].
[43] Parsee A, Haines K, Gallagher S, et al. Cholecystectomy or not? That is the question: analysis of gallbladder pathology in bariatric surgery patients. Presented at Digestive Disorders Week: Society for Surgery of the Alimentary Tract. Chicago, May 14–18, 2005.
[44] Machado M, Marques-Vidal P, Cortez-Pinto H. Hepatic histology in obese patients undergoing bariatric surgery. J Hepatol 2006;45:600–6.
[45] Angulo P, Keach JC, Batts KP, et al. Independent predictors of liver fibrosis in patients with nonalcoholic steatohepatitis. Hepatology 1999;30:1356–62.
[46] Silverman JF, O'Brien KF, Long S, et al. Liver pathology in morbidly obese patients with and without diabetes. Am J Gastroenterol 1990;85:1349–55.
[47] Saadeh S, Younossi ZM, Remer EM, et al. The utility of radiological imaging in nonalcoholic fatty liver disease. Gastroenterology 2002;123:745–50.
[48] Shalhub S, Parsee A, Gallagher SF, et al. The importance of routine liver biopsy in diagnosing nonalcoholic steatohepatitis in bariatric patients. Obes Surg 2004;14:54–9.
[49] Requarth JA, Burchard KW, Colacchio TA, et al. Long-term morbidity following jejunoileal bypass: the continuing potential need for surgical reversal. Arch Surg 1995;130:318–25.
[50] Dixon JB, Bhathal PS, Hughes NR, et al. Nonalcoholic fatty liver disease: improvement in liver histological analysis with weight loss. Hepatology 2004;39:1647–54.
[51] Kral JG, Thung SN, Biron S, et al. Effects of surgical treatment of the metabolic syndrome on liver fibrosis and cirrhosis. Surgery 2004;135:48–58.
[52] Hoeger K. Obesity and weight loss in polycystic ovary syndrome. Obstet Gynecol Clin North Am 2001;28:85–97, vi-vii.
[53] The Rotterdam ESHRE/ASRM-sponsored PCOS Consensus Workshop Group. Revised 2003 consensus on diagnostic criteria and long-term health risks related to polycystic ovary syndrome (PCOS). Hum Reprod 2004;19:41–7.
[54] Eid GM, Cottam DR, Velcu LM, et al. Effective treatment of polycystic ovarian syndrome with Roux-en-Y gastric bypass. Surg Obes Relat Dis 2005;1:77–80.
[55] Buchwald H, Avidor Y, Braunwald E, et al. Bariatric surgery: a systematic review and meta-analysis. Jama 2004;292:1724–37.
[56] Flum DR, Dellinger EP. Impact of gastric bypass operation on survival: a population-based analysis. J Am Coll Surg 2004;199:543–51.
[57] Brodsky JB, Lemmens HJ, Brock-Utne JG, et al. Morbid obesity and tracheal intubation. Anesth Analg 2002;94:732–6.
[58] Ogunnaike BO, Jones SB, Jones DB, et al. Anesthetic considerations for bariatric surgery. Anesth Analg 2002;95:1793–805.
[59] Pieracci FM, Barie PS, Pomp A. Critical care of the bariatric patient. Crit Care Med 2006;34: 1796–804.

ELSEVIER
SAUNDERS

THE MEDICAL
CLINICS
OF NORTH AMERICA

Med Clin N Am 91 (2007) 353–381

Bariatric Surgery Primer for the Internist: Keys to the Surgical Consultation

Daniel Leslie, MD*, Todd A. Kellogg, MD,
Sayeed Ikramuddin, MD

*Section of Gastrointestinal Surgery, Department of Surgery,
University of Minnesota, Minneapolis, MN 55455, USA*

The National Health and Nutrition Examination Survey indicates that the prevalence of obesity defined as a body mass index (BMI) ≥ 30 kg/m^2 for all adults aged 20 or greater in the United States has increased from 13.4% in 1960–1962 to 32.2% in 2003–2004. The study also shows a 4.8% prevalence of adults (2.8% men and 6.9% women) with BMI ≥ 40 kg/m^2. This represents about 14.4 million adults in the United States with morbid obesity on the basis of BMI alone [1,2]. Bariatric surgery is the most effective method for achieving sustained weight loss of considerable degree in individuals with morbid obesity. As a result of the increasing prevalence of morbid obesity, the increasing and improved physician awareness of treating obesity and its attendant medical and psychosocial morbidities, development of less-invasive techniques for treating morbid obesity, and overall public awareness, the number of bariatric operations performed annually has grown exponentially [3]. Moreover, currently there is no drug on the horizon with any potential to be as effective as surgery in controlling morbid obesity. By way of introduction, it is important to realize that, by itself, surgical management of morbid obesity is not an appropriate treatment. Rather, it must be used in conjunction with lifestyle modification with an emphasis on consistent exercise and dietary moderation.

For these reasons, all physicians need to have some awareness about bariatric surgical operations. It has become increasingly apparent that an improved knowledge set is imperative for the nonsurgeons who are taking care of bariatric patients. In a recent survey of Connecticut primary care physicians, only one in four family practitioners recognizes that the gastric bypass resolves or significantly improves diabetes and about two thirds of

* Corresponding author.
E-mail address: lesli002@umn.edu (D. Leslie).

0025-7125/07/$ - see front matter © 2007 Elsevier Inc. All rights reserved.
doi:10.1016/j.mcna.2007.02.004   *medical.theclinics.com*

physicians who returned surveys incorrectly understand the mortality rate from obesity surgery to be more than four times higher than recognized mortality rates [4]. Moreover, media influences exert tremendous power through anecdotal examples of tremendous weight loss by richly rewarded subjects who are taken from several standard deviations away from the mean. Unfortunately, these patients do not represent the average patient and an understanding of obesity through sound bite and video clip causes misperception of scientific reality.

To understand best how to obtain surgical consultation for bariatric surgery, a physician must have an understanding of the role of laparoscopy in obesity surgery, a grasp of the different types of operations available for morbid obesity, and a clear view of the more recent systems-based approach to treating bariatric patients in centers of excellence, which use high-volume providers working in high-volume hospitals.

Advantages of laparoscopy

Advances in laparoscopic skills and instrumentation have enabled surgeons to perform all of the operations for morbid obesity laparoscopically. The goal of the laparoscopic approach, similar to other minimally invasive operations, is to reduce postoperative pain, decrease complications, shorten duration of hospital stay, and return the patient to work and other functional states earlier postoperatively. Laparoscopy achieves the same anatomic objectives as open bariatric surgery but avoids a large abdominal incision. This provides numerous clear benefits: (1) improvement in respiratory mechanics and, therefore, pulmonary function, (2) minimal operative trauma that leads to decreased systemic stress and less pain, and (3) decreased incisional hernia and wound infection risk postoperatively. These effects translate to shorter hospital stay and a faster return to activities of daily living and a lower burden to society from time off.

Pulmonary function

It is well known that major abdominal surgery causes decreased pulmonary function, and this is especially true of upper abdominal surgery [5]. This alteration in pulmonary function leads to respiratory insufficiency and pneumonia in some patients. Improvements in pulmonary function have been shown previously for both laparoscopic cholecystectomy and laparoscopic colectomy compared with their respective open approaches [6–9]. In one study comparing a prospective group of patients undergoing either laparoscopic or open cholecystectomy, marked differences in pulmonary physiology were apparent immediately after surgery. Postoperative functional vital capacity (52% versus 73%, $P = .002$) and forced expiratory volume in 1 second (FEV$_1$) (53% versus 72%, $P = .006$) was markedly reduced in open versus laparoscopic operations [8].

One randomized study of open versus laparoscopic Roux-en-Y gastric bypass (RYGB) documents pulmonary function in 36 patients who underwent laparoscopic RYGB and 34 patients who underwent open RYGB. The overall baseline characteristics of each group were similar and preoperative pulmonary function as measured by forced vital capacity (FVC), FEV$_1$, predicted FEV$_1$, FEV25%–75%, peak expiratory flow (PEF), and maximal ventilatory volume (MVV) were all similar. On postoperative day 1, all patients had marked reduction in all spirometry measures, but the reduction was more profound in patients who underwent open Roux-en-Y gastric bypass ($P < .05$). Specifically, FVC, FEV$_1$, FEV25%–75%, and PEF measured in the 52% to 54% range for the laparoscopic group compared with 39% to 41% for the open group. These differences extended for several of the parameters through at least postoperative day 7 [10].

Although there are clear measurable differences in the mechanics of respiration, these differences have not produced a statistically significant reduction in pneumonia or overall respiratory complications when the laparoscopic approach has been used compared with the open approach in the few randomized, controlled trials available. Moreover, when collected case series are pooled with laparoscopic and open approaches, a difference exists, but it is again not statistically significant (Table 1).

Table 1
Pooled results of complications from controlled and all studies for bariatric procedures

Complication	Controlled trials		All studies	
	Open	Laparoscopic	Open	Laparoscopic
Respiratory	3.0%	1.9%	2.4%	1.5%
Pneumonia	NR	NR	0.9%	0.8%
Medical	NR	NR	6.0%	3.1%
Surgical, preventable and nonpreventable	31.1%	26.1%	22.1%	12.4%
Wound, all	13.1%	0.0%	11.4%[a]	2.3%
Major wound infection	3.0%	0.0%	4.0%[a]	1.6%
Minor wound infection	14.3%	0.0%	10.8%[a]	3.3%
Incisional hernia	8.2%	0.0%	11.9%[a]	0.4%
Internal hernia	0.0%	1.3%	1.4%	2.9%
Splenic injury	NR	NR	1.2%	0.2%
Reoperation	0.0%	4.0%	8.1%	2.7%
Deep venous thrombosis, pulmonary embolus, or both	1.0%	0.9%	1.3%	0.6%

Ninety-eight studies of open procedure and 53 studies of laparoscopic procedure; procedure type not specified.

Abbreviation: NR, not reported.

[a] Statistically significant difference ($P < .05$) between open and laparoscopic approach.

Adapted from Maggard MA, Shugarman LR, Suttorp M, et al. Meta-analysis: surgical treatment of obesity. Ann Intern Med 2005;142(7):547–59; with permission.

Systemic stress and postoperative pain

The laparoscopic approach has been shown to reduce organ system impairment. The hypermetabolic stress response to surgery, which can be characterized by increased energy expenditure, myocardial O_2 demand, pulmonary workload, and renal workload starts with tissues injury and has a direct or indirect affect on most organ systems, which leads to higher perioperative morbidity. The overall stress response is directly proportional to the magnitude of tissue injury. The hypermetabolic response, which can be tested by measuring plasma catecholamines, cortisol, glucose, cytokines, and other acute-phase reactants, is reduced after laparoscopic surgery compared with open surgery [11]. Cell-mediated immunity is also not impaired to the same degree after laparoscopic compared with open surgery [12]. In conjunction with a randomized, controlled study of open versus laparoscopic gastric bypass, systemic stress response was examined. Although some of the markers of the systemic stress response were similar between the two groups of patients, norepinephrine, adrenocorticotropic hormone, C-reactive protein, and interleukin-6 (IL-6) concentrations were all lower after laparoscopic surgery compared with the open counterpart operation, which suggest a measurably lower extent of operative injury [13].

Incisional hernia risk and wound infection

The access laparotomy incision contributes to perioperative morbidity and postoperative recovery time. Open bariatric operations require extended incisions in patients with relatively advanced comorbidities. Therefore, a laparoscopic approach for these patients provides the potential for greater reduction in relative risk compared with healthy low-risk patients who undergo laparotomy. Previous open gastric bypass series have shown an incisional hernia risk between 0.0 and 23.9% [14], and a meta-analysis of obesity procedures showed an 11.9% incisional hernia risk, statistically greater than the 0.4% risk associated with the laparoscopic approach [15]. Management of these hernias postoperatively adds substantially to the overall postoperative cost on these patients. It is preferable for the patient to avoid postoperative incisional hernia despite the justification that it may facilitate insurance coverage for an elective panniculectomy. Management of hernias is not benign and can carry a significant attendant morbidity of seromas and fistula formation.

Though there is a remarkable difference in the incisional hernia rate for open and laparoscopic gastric bypass, an important issue with respect to weight reduction surgery must be emphasized. Obesity surgery performed in either open or laparoscopic fashion is an excellent way to decrease the risk of recurrence in this population.

Surgical site infection (SSI) also occurs at a significantly higher rate in patients who undergo open compared with laparoscopic bariatric surgery. In the randomized, controlled trials available, the incidence of all types of wound infections was 0.0% for the laparoscopic approach and 13.1% for the open approach, and major wound infections occurred in 3.0%. Examination of multiple noncontrolled studies showed a similar difference that was statistically significant for all wounds considered together (2.3% versus 11.4%) and for all major wound infections considered separately (1.6% versus 4.0%).

In obese patients, SSIs are not easily treated, and they can be quite costly. Long-term sequelae include an increase in the incidence of ventral incisional hernia formation. The treatment pathway usually requires a re-admission to the hospital with initiation of intravenous antibiotics. Occasionally, the patient will require an operative procedure, though most of the time they can be treated at bedside. For deep surgical site infections, computed tomography–guided aspiration of intra-abdominal abscess is required. Though patients with SSI are discharged from the hospital earlier now, in most cases extensive outpatient therapy with home health nursing visits and wound vacuum assist closure (VAC) devices are required. One recent estimate for the cost of using home health nurses to treat SSI after elective colorectal surgery is $6200 per case [16]. Wound infections in morbidly obese patients are typically larger and require a longer duration of home health nursing to treat the SSI compared with the patient population in this recent estimate. Moreover, they are more likely to require costly VAC devices.

Morbid obesity operations

The first operation specifically for morbid obesity, jejunoileal bypass, was documented by Kremen and colleagues [17] in Minneapolis, Minnesota in 1954. Since that time, many operations have been developed for the treatment of morbid obesity, but only a few have been considered successful. A successful obesity operation has three main goals: (1) significant magnitude and duration of weight loss, (2) resolution or amelioration of comorbidities related to obesity, and (3) a reasonably low perioperative and long-term complication rate.

Operative techniques for treating morbid obesity are comprised of two categories: restrictive and malabsorptive procedures (or a combination of both). The restrictive procedures, which include the laparoscopic adjustable gastric band and the vertical banded gastroplasty (VBG), are usually simple, technically straightforward operations with low morbidity and mortality. Currently, indications for the VBG are rare. It is suggested that the VBG ultimately fails to be effective in the long term, and Medicare no longer pays for this procedure [18,19]. The restrictive component of the operation is produced by banding the gastric outlet via placement of a foreign body such as a Silastic (Dow Corning, Midland, Michigan) ring, an adjustable silicone band, or prosthetic mesh. Patient cooperation is required to maintain a restricted diet and avoid forced overfeeding and frequent vomiting.

Inappropriate diet from binging or emesis enlarges the proximal stomach and might damage the restrictive device, which renders the procedure non-functional. Restrictive procedures are only effective in reducing the volume of solid food consumed by the patient. Liquid and semisolid, high-calorie foods can often pass through the banded outlet without creating a sense of satiety, which enables some patients to maintain or regain the excessive weight. These procedures are less likely to succeed for the treatment of morbidly obese sweet eaters.

Combined restrictive/malabsorptive operations are the most commonly performed in the United States, and the model is the RYGB. These operations combine excellent restriction by creating a very small gastric pouch with a small distal outlet into the Roux limb of jejunum with mild malabsorption by bypassing a segment of small intestine (75–150 cm).

The malabsorptive obesity procedure produces a controlled state of malabsorption by reducing the contact of digested food with secretions from the liver, pancreas, small bowel, or a combination of these. In theory, a patient with this form of operation should be able to eat an unrestricted diet and still lose weight. The prototype operation in this group was the jejunoileal bypass, which has been abandoned because of liver complications. The duodenal switch is now the model malabsorptive procedure, although there is also a small degree of restriction created by performing a partial gastrectomy to create a narrow gastric tube. These are complex, technically challenging procedures that fundamentally alter the anatomy of the gastrointestinal tract. Occasionally, the amount of malabsorption is unpredictable, and malnutrition occurs, which necessitates reoperation and modification of the original procedure.

The internist should have a clear understanding of the four most commonly discussed operations for morbid obesity at this time: (1) laparoscopic Roux-en-Y gastric bypass (LRYGB), (2) laparoscopic adjustable gastric banding (LAGB), (3) duodenal switch (DS), and (4) laparoscopic sleeve gastrectomy (LSG).

Currently, the two most common procedures being performed for morbid obesity are LRYGB and LAGB. Wittgrove and colleagues [20] described the first LRYGB in 1994, and it is currently the most commonly performed procedure for morbid obesity in the United States (RYGB, both open and laparoscopic, accounted for 80% of all bariatric procedures in the United States in 2002) [21]. Adjustable gastric banding was first performed by Kuzmak [22] in 1986 using an open technique and, with the advent of rapid advances in laparoscopic techniques, was converted to a laparoscopic approach by Belachew and colleagues [23] in September 1993. The DS operation was developed by Hess and Hess [24] and Marceau and colleagues [25] as a hybrid operation, combining the biliopancreatic diversion as described by Scopinaro and colleagues [26] in 1979 and the Demeester and colleagues [27] DS, which was developed to treat and prevent bile reflux. From a laparoscopic standpoint, the DS is highly technically challenging, but it is being performed commonly by a few centers [28]. More often, this operation is being performed using a standard laparotomy incision. The LSG is slowly gaining a niche as a first-stage procedure for super morbidly obese patients with multiple medical risk factors for whom a second-stage procedure involving several anastomoses can be made safer after weight loss and comorbidity resolution.

To understand how to appropriately refer patients for obesity surgery, it is useful to first understand how patients are chosen, how each procedure is performed, what postoperative issues exist, and what complications and long-term results are expected. This review has not considered operations that have been disproven or superceded, eg, jejunoileal bypass, loop gastric bypass, and vertical banded gastroplasty.

Procedure selection

After a patient has undergone a thorough preoperative workup, consideration for the appropriate choice of operation begins with a full assessment of patient expectations, an understanding of how history and physical examination apply to the surgical procedure, laboratory data, and appropriate imaging and endoscopic studies.

After fully understanding the expected risks and benefits of proceeding with each bariatric surgical option, in the end, each of the procedures is a tool that the patient needs to feel comfortable using. Although the importance of how certain underlying medical conditions will contribute to morbidity or outcome with each surgical option is emphasized, the patient always has the final choice after understanding the advantages and disadvantages (Table 2).

Attempts have been made to construct an algorithm for selecting a best procedure for each patient, but at best this approach is rudimentary and makes too many assumptions to be practical. First, the operative techniques continue to evolve, so there is single gold standard procedure. In addition, not all bariatric surgeons perform all bariatric procedures. Finally, there are typically enough differences between each patient population that it is difficult to match each patient with a different operation [29].

Super obese patients are better suited for DS or RYGB procedures. Super-super obese individuals with marked comorbidity are considered for sleeve gastrectomy because it is technically less complicated, and there is no gastrointestinal anastomosis. Patients with cravings for sweet carbohydrate-rich foods probably benefit from operations that provide a negative biofeedback after eating sweets such as the gastric bypass. Need for endoscopic surveillance of the stomach is a contraindication for gastric bypass, whereas patients with a long-term need for nonsteroidal anti-inflammatory drugs because of severe rheumatoid arthritis probably benefit from the duodenal switch, which is nonulcerogenic.

Laparoscopic adjustable gastric banding (LAGB), also known as the LAP-BAND (Allergan Inamed, Santa Barbara, California), contributed to

Table 2
Advantages and disadvantages of different laparoscopic bariatric procedures

Laparoscopic procedure	Advantages	Disadvantages
Vertical banded Gastroplasty	No intestinal anastomosis	Foreign body
	No malabsorption	High long-term failure rate
		No longer approved by Medicare
Adjustable gastric banding	Technically simple	Foreign body
	Low morbidity and mortality	15%–30% failure rate
	Removable	May promote maladaptive eating behavior
	No intestinal anastomosis	
	No malabsorption	
Roux-en-Y gastric bypass	Sustained weight loss	Intestinal anastomosis
	Dumping in sweet eaters	Loss of access to gastric remnant
	Resolution of gastroesophageal reflux disease	Mild risk of vitamin deficiencies
		Marginal ulceration
Duodenal Switch	Excellent sustained weight loss	Technically demanding
	Larger portion size	Frequent bowel movements and flatulence
	No marginal ulcers	Protein and vitamin deficiencies
Sleeve Gastrectomy	Technically simple	May require second-stage procedure
	Low morbidity	Unknown long-term results

the worldwide exponential boom of obesity surgery in the late 1990s. The procedure is technically simple, early results were comparable with those of other restrictive bariatric operations, morbidity was very low, and mortality was nearly nonexistent. A number of enthusiastic surgeons, especially in Australia, Europe, and Latin America published large series and adopted the LAP-BAND as the procedure of choice for morbid obesity and published large series. Because this is the only obesity procedure dependent on a manufactured "device," US Food and Drug Administration approval was finally granted in 2001, so gastric banding has been less common in the United States until recently.

There are two main appeals from a surgical standpoint in performing LAGB: (1) it is technically easy, which makes the operation achievable by most general surgeons in most patients and (2) the absence of intestinal anastomosis removes a disastrous complication from the risks for the morbidly obese patient.

The operation to place an adjustable gastric band is started similar to LRYGB with carbon dioxide pneumoperitoneum, five or six ports, and a liver retractor device. One of the ports must be 15 mm in size to fit the band. The surgeon begins the operation by taking down peritoneal attachments at the angle of His, exposing the left crus, and separating crus from cardia and fundus. Then the lesser sac is entered on the lesser curvature side of the stomach, and the right crus is identified underneath the esophagus. A pathway posterior to the esophagus and adjacent but inferior to the right and left crus is established with a grasper. This position for the band is called the pars flaccida technique.

The band and catheter is prepared and passed through the 15-mm port into the abdomen. It is passed around the upper stomach and locked into place. Several interrupted stitches are applied to gastric tissue across the band to fix the band in place (Fig. 1). The abdominal portion of the operation is now complete; the liver retractor is removed, and the catheter from the band is passed out of the abdomen through a trochar site.

The port is now attached to the catheter, and a pocket is formed for the port under the skin, adjacent to the anterior abdominal fascia. The port is secured to the fascia, and the incision is closed in several layers with suture. After securing all skin incisions and applying sterile dressings, the operation is complete. Typically, the port does not undergo its first filling with normal saline for at least 6 to 8 weeks to allow inflammation and swelling at the gastroesophageal junction to recede (Fig. 2).

Using currently accepted techniques and redesigned LAP-BANDs, the world literature supports LAGB as an advantageous operation with acceptable complication rate. Compared with nonoperative treatments such as

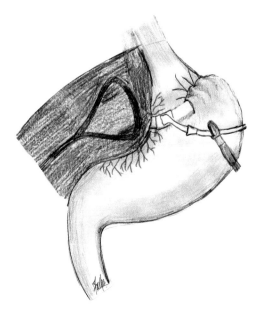

Fig. 1. Laparoscopic adjustable gastric banding.

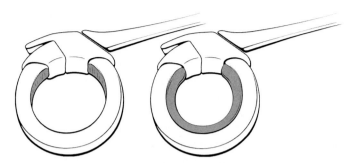

Fig. 2. Gastric band prefilled (left) and filled (right).

dieting and lifestyle modification, LAGB is superior with respect to short-, medium-, and long-term weight loss in available series. Longer-term data are starting to elucidate the potential for excess weight loss, which appears to be about 50% [30]. A number of early adopters of LAGB have published follow-up data exceeding 5 years that has been associated with higher complication rates. Moreover, these investigators have warned that the incidence of complication does not level off several years after surgery; rather, there is a steady increase in complications approaching 3% to 4% per year [31].

Several adjustments to both the surgical technique and engineering of the LAP-BAND device should reduce complication rate in future long-term follow-up series, but these data will not be fully known for several more years. For example, almost all of the bands in the first 5 years were positioned in the perigastric position. This technique has been shown to have a much higher rate of band slippage (with or without pouch dilatation) compared with LAP-BANDs positioned in the pars flaccida location, which is the currently accepted technique (16% versus 4% band prolapse in one prospective study) [32]. Leaking from the system was seen at the connection between the port and catheter, and the manufacturer has now reinforced the connection and lengthened the catheter, which should reduce this complication.

Recently published data from Parikh and colleagues [33] reviewed the experience of one university hospital with gastric banding over a 3-year time period, and they performed immediate postoperative and annual esophagograms on every patient. Of 749 patients studied, 28 (3.7%) experienced early complications within 30 days of band placement. An additional 76 (10.1%) patients experienced late complications, and gastric prolapse or band "slip" occurred in 22 (2.9%) with gastric pouch dilatation without band "slip" occurred in 15 (2.0%) patients. Unrecognized hiatal hernia before operation or development of hiatal hernia after LAP-BAND placement may have contributed to these complications. All patients required revisional surgery to correct the band position or pouch dilatation. Overall in this series, 80 patients (10.7%) required reoperation, and, of these, 46 patients (6.1%) required revision or replacement of the band.

Several complications of the LAP-BAND operation are unlikely to be reduced by surgical technique or band reengineering. Band erosion may ultimately question the durability of LAGB as a procedure for morbid obesity and has been seen now up to 5 years after band placement. Unfortunately, the complication often is asymptomatic, associated only with mild abdominal discomfort and possibly weight regain. Several groups have looked for this complication using surveillance upper endoscopy and have found it in 7.5% to 11.1% of asymptomatic band patients [33,34]. Band erosion causes a dense inflammatory reaction with distortion of tissues at the level of the cardia, leading to technically demanding and complicated reoperative surgery.

The incidence of reflux esophagitis associated with food intolerance has also been very high in some long-term series [31,35]; the treatment of esophagitis is usually to empty the band, which improves the symptomatic food intolerance and reflux esophagitis, but this process leads to weight regain. Replacement of band fluid leads to reduplication of esophagitis and food intolerance, so ultimately the solution for this long-term complication will involve band removal and possibly conversion to a different obesity operation. There is a vigorous tissue reaction that creates a scar at the gastroesophageal location during the time that the band is in position. Therefore, it is far easier to remove the band than to truly reverse the band.

The most important factor in successful long-term outcomes for LAGB is likely to be careful multidisciplinary follow-up. Band adjustment strategies and compliance with dietary restrictions and physical activity are critical to weight loss success, and these vary throughout the United States and the world. Little clinical research has focused on the critical component of band adjustment. Short-term clinical experience with the LAP-BAND in the United States suggests that the device is a safe and effective treatment for morbid obesity, and these results are starting to mirror outcomes from Australia, Europe, and South America [36].

Finally, there are several groups of patients who might not be served well by the LAGB: super-obese patients (who might be better served by DS or LRYGB), patients with type 2 diabetes (in whom diabetes resolution occurs at a higher rate in LRYGB or DS), patients with hiatal hernia or severe gastroesophageal reflux disease (LRYGB is best option), and African-Americans [37]. Patients who might be better served with LAGB are those with a history of peptic ulcer disease.

Laparoscopic Roux-en-Y gastric bypass LRYGB is one of the most difficult and challenging laparoscopic procedures routinely performed today, and it evolved from the open RYGB. The gastric bypass was initially conceived by Mason and Ito [38] as a large gastric pouch drained by a loop gastrojejunostomy connected to the pouch. The procedure evolved in 1977 when Griffen and colleagues [39] suggested using a Roux-en-Y gastrojejunostomy to minimize bile reflux. Other modifications have included fully dividing the stomach pouch from the lower stomach remnant to prevent gastrogastric fistulae. The most dramatic advancement for this procedure was the initial use of laparoscopic technique in 1994, which reduced perioperative morbidity markedly. This approach to bariatric surgery has helped fuel the exponential rise in bariatric procedures performed worldwide over the last 10 years. Gastric bypass combines elements of both restriction, by creating a small stomach, and malabsorption, by bypassing intestine, though the most common lengths of intestine bypassed (100 to 250 cm) should not provide any real long-term nutrient malabsorption.

The technical details of the operation are complex but can be understood readily by dividing the operation into three phases: (1) creation of a very small gastric pouch, (2) construction of the jejunojejunostomy, and (3) construction of the gastrojejunostomy (Fig. 3).

The operation begins with the establishment of pneumoperitoneum using carbon dioxide. A total of five or six laparoscopic ports are placed, and a liver retractor device is used to provide adequate visualization of the upper stomach. The surgeon then starts the operation by creating a 15- 30-mL gastric pouch (a golf ball has a volume of 40 mL) using a laparoscopic cutting staple device across the stomach from lesser curve to cardia. The pouch is completely separated from the gastric remnant, but the remnant is not removed.

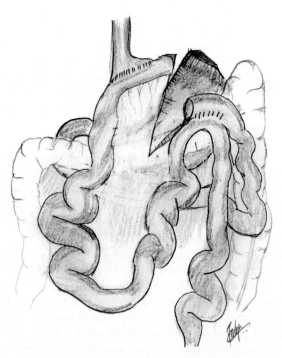

Fig. 3. Laparoscopic Roux-en-Y gastric bypass.

The jejunojejunostomy is started by identifying the ligament of Treitz, and the bowel is then measured 100 cm distally and divided using a cutting stapler device. This creates a distal biliopancreatic limb and a proximal Roux limb. The Roux limb is measured an additional 150 cm distally, and at this location a jejunojejunostomy is constructed between the Roux limb and distal biliopancreatic limb. This is commonly stapled using a laparoscopic stapling device but can also be performed using a hand-sewn method. An antiobstruction stitch is placed to prevent the Roux limb from kinking on itself, and the mesenteric defect is then closed with suture.

The gastrojejunostomy is then constructed by bringing the proximal Roux limb adjacent to the gastric pouch. There are numerous safe and effective ways to create this anastomosis, and surgeons use a technique that has proven safe for them. The gastrojejunostomy anastomosis is then tested for leaks under saline, and the operation is complete.

The altered anatomy produces reliably altered gut absorption, and many patients experience symptoms of dumping syndrome in response to high-calorie sweets intake. This side effect of RYGB is an important difference from purely restrictive operations for morbid obesity and probably explains the greater weight loss achieved with RYGB. Long-term follow-up data exist for the gastric bypass, and its sustained weight loss of approximately 70% [30] combined with a relatively tolerable side effect profile makes LRYGB the gold standard operation for the treatment of morbid obesity.

The technical aspects of this operation and its altered anatomy provide a predictable array of complications in morbidly obese individuals. The most common complication is stenosis of the gastrojejunal anastomosis, which occurs in about 5% of patients and is readily treated with endoscopic dilatation. Patients with this complication complain of diet intolerance within several weeks of surgery, but the cause is not clear. There does not appear to be a relationship to technique of gastrojejunostomy, whether hand sewn or stapled.

The second most common complication has been an increased risk of internal hernia with laparoscopic RYGB. Maggard and colleagues published a meta-analysis that documented a nearly twofold increase in internal hernia for the laparoscopic approach compared with the open RYGB (2.9% versus 1.4%) [15], though this difference was not statistically significant. This difference was likely magnified by several issues in the early case series of LRYGB, which showed this difference: (1) many surgeons did not close any of the internal hernia defects in early series of laparoscopic gastric bypass, and (2) most surgeons initially performed a retrocolic Roux-en-Y anastomosis, which resulted in a third internal hernia defect site and arguably the most common site for internal hernias after laparoscopic gastric bypass [40]. Minimally invasive surgeons have since fashioned operations with a lower internal hernia rate by closing the jejunojejunostomy mesenteric defect and by placing the Roux limb in an antecolic position, which eliminates the retrocolic defect entirely [41,42]. In a recent review of 1400 consecutive cases by one group of surgeons who performed LRYGB in the antecolic, antegastric position, only three internal hernias were documented for a rate of 0.2%. Their operation was performed without division of the mesentery, which reduces the size of the potential space for hernia defects to enter [41]. Moreover, laparoscopic re-exploration of a patient with small bowel obstruction can be performed to diagnose and correct the problem of internal hernia in many cases [43].

The other major complications in the early postoperative period are gastrojejunal anastomotic leak, deep venous thrombosis and pulmonary embolism, and bleeding (Fig. 4). Other major disadvantages of gastric bypass are related to the malabsorptive component of the operation, which results in vitamin deficiencies and reduced bone density. Iron is predominantly absorbed by the duodenum, and because this portion of the gastrointestinal tract is bypassed, iron deficiency is estimated to be between 6% and 33%

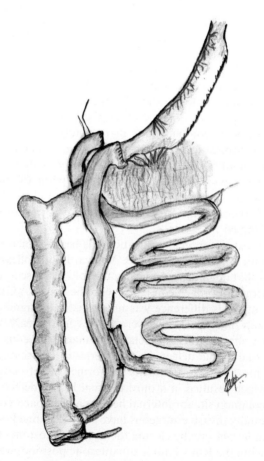

Fig. 4. Laparoscopic duodenal switch.

[44]. Vitamin B12 is deficient in up to 37% and folate in 22% of patients at 2 years' follow-up [45]. The duodenum and proximal jejunum are primary locations for absorption of calcium; therefore, hypocalcemia is a very common postgastric bypass vitamin deficiency. Malabsorption of vitamin D contributes further to calcium malabsorption because gastrointestinal calcium absorption is dependent on vitamin D. Supplementation of each of these mineral and vitamin deficiencies (iron, vitamin B12, folate, and calcium) must be provided in the patient's diet for the rest of their life.

Finally, the distal gastric remnant cannot be accessed directly using standard endoscopic techniques in the event that gastric or duodenal polyps require surveillance or the patient requires urgent endoscopic retrograde cholangiopancreatography (ERCP). For this reason, patients who have known polyps seen on upper endoscopy should not undergo LRYGB; they might be better suited for LAGB or DS. The gastric remnant can be accessed safely to facilitate performance of ERCP by a combined laparoscopic and endoscopic operation. A gastrostomy tube is left in place for further manipulations.

Laparoscopic duodenal switch

The DS procedure has greater technical complexity (particularly when performed laparoscopically) and greater perceived perioperative and nutritional risks in comparison with RYGB. This has limited the widespread adoption of DS among bariatric surgeons. Nonetheless, two recent meta-analyses suggest that weight loss results after DS may be superior to those in RYGB [15,46], and at least one retrospective series has shown excellent outcomes at 10 years or more [47].

This operation is more challenging technically than LRYGB and is also logically separated into three components: (1) creation of a gastric sleeve, (2) construction of a duodenoileostomy (alimentary limb), and (3) construction of the ileoileostomy (see Fig. 4).

The operation begins with insufflation of the abdomen using carbon dioxide. Six laparoscopic ports and the liver retractor device are placed. A 200- 500-mL gastric sleeve is created by sequentially firing laparoscopic linear cutting stapler devices from a point 6 cm proximal to the pylorus on the greater curvature to the angle of His next to the gastroesophageal junction. This is performed with a Bougie dilator in place to appropriately size the gastric sleeve. The greater curvature specimen is removed from the abdomen.

The duodenum is then prepared for duodenoileostomy by carefully dissecting and transecting the duodenum 2 to 5 cm past the pylorus. A 150-cm alimentary limb of ileum is prepared by transecting the ileum 250 cm proximal to the ileocecal valve with a linear cutting stapler. This will ultimately fashion a 150-cm alimentary limb and a 100-cm common channel from the distal segment of bowel. The proximal bowel between ligament of Treitz and the staple line is called the biliopancreatic limb. The proximal alimentary limb is then brought through the transverse colon mesentery and anastomosed to the proximal duodenum to construct the duodenoileostomy. The technique of anastomosis can be completely or partially hand sewn or completely stapled. The integrity of this anastomosis can be tested with the gastroscope using air insufflation under normal saline or using an orogastric tube and methylene blue instillation.

The distal ileoileostomy anastomosis approximates the end of the biliopancreatic limb to the alimentary limb 100 cm above the ileocecal valve and can also be performed using staplers or sutures. The mesenteric defects created by the bowel reconfiguration are closed to prevent internal herniation.

The malabsorption anatomy created by the duodenal switch is defined by the lengths of each limb. The operation described above results in a 150-cm alimentary limb and a 100-cm common channel and a biliopancreatic limb that is much longer but not measured. Numerous other methods are used to configure the length of each limb, but a common denominator is the use of a common channel length between 50 and 100 cm. The limb lengths are used as a proxy for a measurement of the total surface area of each portion of bowel, which is more accurately determined by the microstructural contributions of the brush border and villi, among other factors [28].

The altered gastrointestinal configuration provided by DS results in rapid weight loss through a predominantly malabsorptive mechanism. The excess weight loss remains consistently at around 70% even after 6 years of follow-up [46]. Complications of the operation are significant. One study of 1150 patients who underwent open DS documented mortality in 0.57%, gastric leaks in 0.7%, revisions in 3.7%, and reversals in 0.61% [47]. Moreover, chronic gastrointestinal symptoms occur in 38% (flatulence and diarrhea), and malabsorption can be a significant problem [15]. Protein deficiency has been a major concern in DS, and hypoalbuminemia has been reported in up to 18% of patients at 28 months when a common channel length of 50 cm was used [48]; in a different study of 589 patients in which the common channel was 100 cm, albumin and total protein levels remained within normal limits up to 3 years postoperatively [49]. Moreover, vitamin B12, calcium, and all of the fat-soluble vitamins are frequently deficient after DS and require chronic supplementation [44].

Laparoscopic sleeve gastrectomy

As bariatric surgery has grown rapidly and referring physicians have become more aware of the beneficial outcomes, increasingly complicated cases are being referred for major operative therapy, which comes with concomitant high risk for these patients. The specific group of severely obese individuals with BMI >60 kg/m^2, life-threatening comorbidity, and extremely poor quality of life have a very high potential for benefit from bariatric surgery. Unfortunately, they also represent the highest-risk patient for undergoing bariatric repair, with mortality rates markedly higher than their lower-risk morbidly obese counterparts with BMI 35 to 60 kg/m^2, fewer co-morbidities, and better quality of life [50,51].

Bariatric surgeons have advocated for a two-stage obesity procedure that includes a safer, less-invasive preliminary stage followed by a completion operation after the patient has lost a large amount of their excess weight [52–54]. The sleeve gastrectomy is one approach that is being studied now and can be performed laparoscopically. This involves a longitudinal resection of the fundus, body, and antrum leaving a stomach tube conduit based on the lesser curve (Fig. 5). The procedure is effective and flexible, providing an option for conversion to DS or RYGB or, in some individuals, may serve as the final weight loss operation. Unfortunately, the sleeve gastrectomy has not yet been universally accepted as an operation for morbid obesity because long-term data are lacking. Third-party payors often are willing to pay for the operation, but this typically requires a prolonged period of documentation and preauthorization approval.

In a study performed at the University of Pittsburgh by Cottam and colleagues [54], 126 patients with mean BMI of 65.3 (range, 45 to 91) and most with American Society of Anesthesiologists (ASA) score of III or IV,

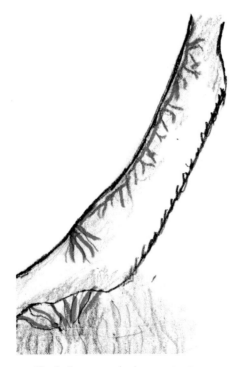

Fig. 5. Laparoscopic sleeve gastrectomy.

underwent LSG as a first-stage operation. These patients had an average of 9.3 comorbidities each. At 12 months' follow-up, mean excess weight loss was 46%, and there was one distant mortality and a 13% incidence of major complications. A subgroup of 36 patients with excess weight loss of 38%, decreased ASA score in almost all, and significantly reduced number of co-morbidities were revised subsequently with a second-stage procedure to LRYGB. There was no mortality and an 8% incidence of major complication.

From a technical standpoint, the sleeve gastrectomy provides several major benefits. In most cases, the operation can be performed laparoscopically, which mitigates postoperative stress and recovery for the patient. Moreover, there are no gastrointestinal anastomoses, and this reduces the probability of a gastrointestinal leak and associated higher risk of death in an otherwise high-risk patient population. The LSG has no long-term sequelae when left in place. The role of LSG as a primary operation for morbid operation requires further study [54].

Considerations of surgeon volume and facility volume

The relationship between surgical volume and mortality has been a subject of intense scrutiny over the last 25 years [55–57]. Now in the era of an extremely safety- and cost-conscious health care environment, there is also strong interest in regional referral of patients to hospitals and surgical teams that have special expertise treating a given surgical problem.

The treatment of pancreatic cancer at high-volume hospitals by high-volume surgeons is perhaps one of the best early examples of concentrating patients with a surgical diagnosis at one center of excellence. The group at Johns Hopkins found a much higher mortality rate for patients treated by resection for pancreatic cancer when performed by low-volume providers compared with medium- and high-volume providers. The relative risk for mortality was 19-fold greater at hospitals with low-volume providers and eightfold higher at hospitals with medium-volume providers. Moreover, hospital length of stay and hospital charge was also markedly elevated at low-volume hospitals compared with a high-volume center [58]. This same concept has been shown to be true with respect to mortality or complications for ruptured and elective abdominal aortic aneurysm repair [59,60], carotid endarterectomy [61], elective colon resection [62], primary and revision hip repairs [63], radical prostatectomy [64], coronary artery bygass graft [65], and treatment of nonruptured intracranial aneurysm [66].

Bariatric surgery, in particular, can carry a substantial risk including death. The preoperative optimization of patients can be demanding, the operations are technically challenging, the postoperative nursing care requires specialty training, and short- and long-term metabolic derangements require focused attention. All of these difficulties can lead to significant morbidity and mortality, yet there have been numerous centers through the United States that have reported excellent results and acceptably low morbidity and very low mortality with different types of obesity operations and with different patient populations. In one series of 1040 morbidly obese patients who underwent LRYGB, Higa and colleagues [67] reported only one 30-day mortality, whereas in a more recent series of 350 super-obese patients (super-obese = BMI ≥ 50 kg/m^2) who underwent laparoscopic duodenal switch or LRYGB, Prachand and his colleagues [28] only reported one mortality.

Scrutiny of outcomes has placed the bariatric medical community in an unusual predicament. Bariatric surgeons were faced with a national obesity epidemic and had a successful treatment available that cures or prevents type 2diabetes along with asthma, hypertension, obstructive sleep apnea, and stress incontinence and provides 60% to 70% of durable excess weight loss. With 140,000 cases being performed annually, obesity surgery is only being offered to 1% of patients who might benefit. At the same time, bariatric surgeons were not able to provide guarantees that all surgeons would deliver safe medical and surgical care to a high-risk population.

Since these events, the ASBS responded by examining a broad set of issues within bariatric surgery aimed at optimizing patient care and achieving continual improvements in quality of care. A comprehensive meta-analysis of the English-language literature from 1990 through 2003 identified 22,094 patients who had undergone bariatric surgery; the excess weight loss was 61.2%, and this was broken down for each type of operation. Moreover, mortality and comorbidity resolution rates were defined (Table 3).

A key component of the reevaluation of bariatric surgery focused on surgeon and hospital volume and its relationship to complication and outcome. The learning curve for LRYGB is steep. Surgeons in one series had a much higher gastrojejunal anastomosis leak rate in their first 50 cases compared with their third 50 cases (10% versus 0%) [68]. Certainly, a number of independent variables contribute to individual surgeon competence in performing these complex procedures, including meticulous technique, technical agility, innate hand-eye coordination, judgment, quality of training, multidisciplinary support, and luck in some situations. However, it is prudent to attempt to limit the number of surgeons climbing this learning curve or at the minimum to make sure each of the surgeons has appropriate mentorship while learning the demanding technical challenges of laparoscopic obesity surgery.

A number of studies have shown that this learning curve leads to real differences in mortality and morbidity when comparing death and adverse events with surgeon and hospital volume for gastric bypass (Table 4). In a population-based study by Courcoulas and colleagues [69], 4674 patients who underwent gastric bypass in Pennsylvania between 1999 and 2001 were reviewed. A total of 73 hospitals and 129 surgeons were involved in these operations. There were 28 deaths in all and 813 adverse outcomes. Surgeons who performed fewer than 10 operations per year (low volume surgeons)

Table 3
Collected outcomes from surgical procedures for morbid obesity

Procedure	EWL	Mortality	Diabetes resolution Resolved	Diabetes resolution Resolved/improved	Improvement in hyperlipidemia Hyperlipidemia	Improvement in hyperlipidemia Hypercholesterolemia	Improvement in hyperlipidemia Hypertriglyceridemia	Hypertension Resolved	Hypertension Resolved/improved	Obstructive sleep apnea Resolved	Obstructive sleep apnea Resolved/improved
Gastric banding	47.5%	0.1%	47.9%	80.8%	71.1%	78.3%	76.9%	43.2%	70.8%	95.0%	68.0%
Gastric bypass	61.6%	0.5%	83.7%	93.2%	93.6%	95.0%	94.1%	67.5%	87.2%	67.5%	87.2%
Biliopancreatic diversion or duodenal switch	70.1%	1.1%	98.9%	76.7%	99.5%	99.7%	100%	83.4%	75.1%	83.4%	75.1%
Total	61.2%		76.8%	86.0%	79.3%	71.3%	82.4%	61.7%	78.5%	85.7%	83.6%

Different numbers of treatment groups were analyzed for each outcome.
Abbreviations: EWL, excess weight loss; Mortality, operative 30-day mortality.
Data from Buchwald H, Avidor Y, Braunwald E, et al. Bariatric surgery: a systematic review and meta-analysis. JAMA 2004;292(14):1724–37.

Table 4
Collected adverse events from surgical procedures for morbid obesity

Procedure	GI symptoms	Reflux	Vomiting	Nutritional and electrolyte abnormalities	Surgical, preventable and not preventable	Anastomotic, gastric pouch or duodenal leak	Anastomotic or stomal stenosis	Bleeding	Reoperation	Medical
LAGB	7.0%	4.7%	2.5%	NR	13.2%	NR	NR	0.3%	7.7	0.7
RYGB	16.9%	10.9%	15.7%	16.9%	18.7%	2.2%	4.6%	2.0%	1.6	4.8
BPD/DS	37.7%	NR	5.9%	NR	5.9%	1.8%	NR	0.2%	4.2	NR

Seventy trials of RYGB, 41 trials of LAGB, and 7 trials of BPD/DS.
Abbreviations: BPD, biliopancreatic diversion; NR, not reported.
Adapted from Maggard MA, Shugarman LR, Suttorp M, et al. Meta-analysis: surgical treatment of obesity. Ann Intern Med 2005;142(7):547–59; with permission.

had a 1.6% mortality rate compared with those who performed more than 100 operations per year (high-volume surgeons) who had a 0.3% mortality rate ($P < .05$). Moreover, 28% of patients experienced adverse events when low-volume surgeons operated compared with 14% when high-volume surgeons operated. These mortality and adverse events rates paralleled the differences in outcome based on the volume of each hospital.

A second study by Nguyen and colleagues [70] examined 24,166 patients who underwent gastric bypass at 93 different academic centers in the United States. Hospitals were separated into low- (<50 cases/year), medium- (50-100 cases/year), and high-volume (>100 cases/year) centers. In low-volume compared with high-volume hospitals, the mortality rate was four times higher (1.2% versus 3.1%, $P < .01$) and when adjusted for expected in-hospital mortality, which adjusts risk on the basis of medical comorbidities, the observed-to-expected in-hospital mortality ratio was still significantly higher at low-volume than high-volume hospitals (3.9% versus 1.2%). Moreover, mean length of hospital stay, overall complications, 30-day readmission rate, and mean cost were all lower when patients underwent operation in high-volume compared with low-volume centers (all $P < .05$).

While the proceeding two studies clearly show a hospital volume-outcome relationship, the true causes for the disparate outcomes is not clear. Volume is more likely a surrogate marker of structural and process components for patient care. Experienced surgeons, nurses, and other health care professionals involved in implementing standardized selection criteria and operative and postoperative care are an important part of the structural component. In addition, hospital-based systems ensure that large wheelchairs, beds, heavy duty operating room tables, and other equipment necessary for the care of the morbidly obese are available. Moreover, these hospital facilities possess diagnostic technology, critical care staffing, and other resources such as rehabilitation facilities appropriately equipped for the care of bariatric patients. Volume is another structural component. Surgeons at high-volume facilities have the ability to refine surgical techniques and thereby improve outcomes. Improvement of the patient selection process and perioperative clinical decision making also leads to a lower rate of medical errors, which has been shown to be associated with increased mortality. The processes of care such as clinical pathways can improve resource use, lower complications, and also reduce in-hospital physician order errors of omission or commission. Taken together, all of these factors likely lead to the improvement in outcome seen at high-volume hospitals [71].

Bariatric surgery, particularly RYGB, is a complex operation performed in a high-risk population with many comorbid conditions. Optimal outcomes in bariatric surgery often depend on the presence of an experienced surgical team working in the context of a well-structured multidisciplinary program. A dedicated surgical team often includes well-trained surgeons, bariatric surgical coordinators, dedicated anesthesiologists, nutritionists, and mental health specialists. A well-structured program includes a hospital facility capable of handling the morbidly obese and the presence of appropriate consultative and critical care staff, experienced nursing staff, perioperative clinical pathways, organized support group, and a clinic system in place for long-term follow-up of patients.

As a result of reviewing the learning curve and in an effort to improve the quality of surgical care for bariatric patients, the American College of Surgeons (ACS) Bariatric Surgery Center Network (BSCN) Accreditation Program and the American Society of Bariatric Surgeons (ASBS) both proposed different methods of accrediting bariatric surgical practices (Table 5 for comparison) [72,73]. The ACS has focused its efforts on dividing bariatric centers into different level designations similar to the designations for trauma hospitals. Level 1 centers would provide complete tertiary care and manage the most challenging and complex patients while level 2 centers would provide care in the setting of a lower volume hospital. A third designation is that of outpatient, and these centers would focus on placement and adjustment of laparoscopic gastric bands.

The ASBS elected to form a private compliance and research organization that functions to accredit bariatric centers on an equal footing. Each of these centers is expected to provide a full spectrum of bariatric surgical care, and there is no difference in qualification from one center to the next.

Criteria for becoming an ASBS-certified "center of excellence" recognize the need for surgeons and hospitals to have adequate yearly volume to offer safe surgical care for patients. Each hospital must have performed at least 125 bariatric surgeries in the preceding 12 months, and each applicant surgeon must have performed at least 125 total bariatric surgeries. At least 50 of them should have occurred in the preceding 12 months. In addition, operative outcomes must be tracked carefully, and complete databases must be kept for all surgeons from the center of excellence.

Summary

The increasing prevalence of morbid obesity in North America combined with the refinement of laparoscopic techniques for the performing these operations has contributed to the exponential growth of bariatric surgery over the last 10 years. There are many important considerations for the internist who is referring a patient for bariatric surgery. First and foremost, there is a clear difference in outcome and safety after laparoscopic compared with open bariatric surgery, and this must be considered carefully in the surgical consultation. Second, there are now at least four complex operations that combat morbid obesity. Although the LRYGB has become the gold standard obesity operation in the United States, there currently are no validated algorithms for selecting an operation for each patient. It is vitally important

Table 5
Comparison of requirements for ACS BSCN and ASBS accreditation requirements

ACS BSCN levels of accreditation program	ASBS Center of excellence requirement of a hospital for provisional status
A total of five designations will be applied: level 1a, level 1b, level 2a, level 2b, and outpatient	There is an institutional commitment at the highest levels of the applicant medical staff and the institution's administration to excellence in the care of bariatric surgical patients as documented with an ongoing regularly scheduled in-service education program in bariatric surgery.
Level 1 centers provide complete tertiary care and devote resources to bariatric surgery. The most challenging and complex patients are managed. All levels of obesity, obesity procedures, ages, comorbid conditions, and revisions will be engaged.	The applicant institution has performed at least 125 bariatric surgical operations in the preceding 12 months, and each applicant surgeon has performed at least 125 total bariatric operations and performed at least 50 operations in the preceding 12 months.
Level 2 centers will be designated for hospitals in which obesity surgery volumes are not as high. It is expected that these centers will perform 25 or more operations annually for weight loss. Surgeons in these centers will have performed 50 or more primary operations for obesity in the past two years.	The applicant maintains a medical director for bariatric surgery who participates in the relevant decision-making administrative meetings of the institution.
Outpatient centers will be credentialed for providing application and adjustment of laparoscopic gastric bands. A credentialed and experienced bariatric surgeon will perform at least 50 primary weight-loss operations annually and the center will also perform 50 or more weight-loss operations annually.	The applicant maintains a full complement of the various consultative services required for the care of bariatric surgical patients including the immediate availability of full in-house critical care services.
Level 1a and 2a centers will use the ACS National Surgical Quality Improvement Program adapted for bariatric surgery and will employ a trained nurse reviewer to collect and submit data	The applicant maintains a full line of equipment and instruments for the care of bariatric surgical patients including furniture, wheelchairs, operating room tables, beds, radiologic facilities, surgical instruments, and other facilities suitable for morbidly obese and super obese patients.
Level 1b, 2b, and outpatient designations will report outcomes data for accreditation purposes only. A nurse from the bariatric surgical service will collect and enter data using an established protocol by the ACS.	The applicant has a bariatric surgeon who spends a significant portion of his or her efforts in the field of bariatric surgery and who has qualified coverage and support for patient care.

Table 5 (*continued*)

ACS BSCN levels of accreditation program	ASBS Center of excellence requirement of a hospital for provisional status
	The applicant uses clinical pathway orders that facilitate the standardization of perioperative care for the relevant procedure. In addition, all bariatric surgical procedures are standardized for each surgeon.
	The applicant uses designated nurses or physician extenders who are dedicated to serving bariatric surgical patients and who are involved in continuing education in the care of bariatric patients.
	The applicant makes available organized and supervised support groups for all patients who have undergone bariatric surgery at the institution. The activities of the support group should be documented, including group locations, meeting times, supervisor, curriculum, and attendance. For example, such activities as on-line chat rooms, Web-based support groups, exercise, instruction, and clothing sales should be noted.
	The applicant provides documentation of a program dedicated to a goal of long-term patient follow-up of at least 75% for bariatric procedures at 5 years with a monitoring and tracking system for outcomes and agrees to provide annual outcome summaries to the SRC in a manner consistent with Health Insurance Portability and Accountability Act of 1996 (HIPAA) regulations.
	The applicant agrees to enter all patients who undergo surgery in the group's or individual practice; no patients will be excluded.

Adapted from American College of Surgeons Bariatric Surgery Center Network Levels of Accreditation. ACS, 2006. (Accessed December 7, 2006, at http://www.facs.org/cqi/bscn/levelsdefined.html.) and Rendon SE, Pories WJ. Quality assurance in bariatric surgery. Surg Clin North Am 2005;85(4):757–71, vi–vii; with permission.

to have a strong understanding of each operation so that postoperative complications can be anticipated and readily treated. Finally, the concept of a bariatric center of excellence only recently has been introduced after years of data have supported the concept of concentrating complex operations in the hands of a few surgeons in the setting of high-volume hospitals.

References

[1] Flegal KM, Carroll MD, Ogden CL, et al. Prevalence and trends in obesity among US adults, 1999–2000. JAMA 2002;288(14):1723–7.
[2] Ogden CL, Carroll MD, Curtin LR, et al. Prevalence of overweight and obesity in the United States, 1999-2004. JAMA 2006;295(13):1549–55.
[3] Steinbrook R. Surgery for severe obesity. N Engl J Med 2004;350(11):1075–9.
[4] Frangou C. Family physicians still wary of bariatric surgery. General Surgery News 2006 September: 1–20.
[5] Latimer RG, Dickman M, Day WC, et al. Ventilatory patterns and pulmonary complications after upper abdominal surgery determined by preoperative and postoperative computerized spirometry and blood gas analysis. Am J Surg 1971;122(5):622–32.
[6] McMahon AJ, Baxter JN, Kenny G, et al. Ventilatory and blood gas changes during laparoscopic and open cholecystectomy. Br J Surg 1993;80(10):1252–4.
[7] Schauer PR, Luna J, Ghiatas AA, et al. Pulmonary function after laparoscopic cholecystectomy. Surgery 1993;114(2):389–97 [discussion: 97–9].
[8] Frazee RC, Roberts JW, Okeson GC, et al. Open versus laparoscopic cholecystectomy. A comparison of postoperative pulmonary function. Ann Surg 1991;213(6):651–3 [discussion: 3–4].
[9] Schwenk W, Bohm B, Witt C, et al. Pulmonary function following laparoscopic or conventional colorectal resection: a randomized controlled evaluation. Arch Surg 1999;134(1):6–12 [discussion: 3].
[10] Nguyen NT, Lee SL, Goldman C, et al. Comparison of pulmonary function and postoperative pain after laparoscopic versus open gastric bypass: a randomized trial. J Am Coll Surg 2001;192(4):469–76 [discussion: 76–7].
[11] Schauer PR, Sirinek KR. The laparoscopic approach reduces the endocrine response to elective cholecystectomy. Am Surg 1995;61(2):106–11.
[12] Allendorf JD, Bessler M, Whelan RL, et al. Postoperative immune function varies inversely with the degree of surgical trauma in a murine model. Surg Endosc 1997;11(5):427–30.
[13] Nguyen NT, Goldman CD, Ho HS, et al. Systemic stress response after laparoscopic and open gastric bypass. J Am Coll Surg 2002;194(5):557–66 [discussion: 66–7].
[14] Schauer PR, Ikramuddin S. Laparoscopic surgery for morbid obesity. Surg Clin North Am 2001;81(5):1145–79.
[15] Maggard MA, Shugarman LR, Suttorp M, et al. Meta-analysis: surgical treatment of obesity. Ann Intern Med 2005;142(7):547–59.
[16] Smith RL, Bohl JK, McElearney ST, et al. Wound infection after elective colorectal resection. Ann Surg 2004;239(5):599–605 [discussion: 7].
[17] Kremen AJ, Linner JH, Nelson CH. An experimental evaluation of the nutritional importance of proximal and distal small intestine. Ann Surg 1954;140(3):439–48.
[18] Balsiger BM, Poggio JL, Mai J, et al. Ten and more years after vertical banded gastroplasty as primary operation for morbid obesity. J Gastrointest Surg 2000;4(6):598–605.
[19] Morinigo R, Moize V, Musri M, et al. Glucagon-like peptide-1, peptide YY, hunger, and satiety after gastric bypass surgery in morbidly obese subjects. J Clin Endocrinol Metab 2006;91(5):1735–40.
[20] Wittgrove AC, Clark GW, Tremblay LJ. Laparoscopic gastric bypass, Roux-en-Y: preliminary report of five cases. Obes Surg 1994;4(4):353–7.
[21] Santry HP, Gillen DL, Lauderdale DS. Trends in bariatric surgical procedures. JAMA 2005;294(15):1909–17.
[22] Kuzmak LI. Silicone gastric banding: a simple and effective operation for morbid obesity. Contemp Surg 1986;28(1):13–8.
[23] Belachew M, Legrand MJ, Defechereux TH, et al. Laparoscopic adjustable silicone gastric banding in the treatment of morbid obesity. A preliminary report. Surg Endosc 1994;8(11):1354–6.

[24] Hess DS, Hess DW. Biliopancreatic diversion with a duodenal switch. Obes Surg 1998;8(3): 267–82.

[25] Marceau P, Hould FS, Simard S, et al. Biliopancreatic diversion with duodenal switch. World J Surg 1998;22(9):947–54.

[26] Scopinaro N, Gianetta E, Civalleri D, et al. Bilio-pancreatic bypass for obesity: II. Initial experience in man. Br J Surg 1979;66(9):618–20.

[27] DeMeester TR, Fuchs KH, Ball CS, et al. Experimental and clinical results with proximal end-to-end duodenojejunostomy for pathologic duodenogastric reflux. Ann Surg 1987; 206(4):414–26.

[28] Prachand VN, Davee RT, Alverdy JC. Duodenal switch provides superior weight loss in the super-obese (BMI > or = 50 kg/m^2) compared with gastric bypass. Ann Surg 2006;244(4): 611–9.

[29] Buchwald H. A bariatric surgery algorithm. Obes Surg 2002;12(6):733–46 [discussion: 47–50].

[30] Van Hee RH. Biliopancreatic diversion in the surgical treatment of morbid obesity. World J Surg 2004;28(5):435–44.

[31] Suter M, Calmes JM, Paroz A, et al. A 10-year experience with laparoscopic gastric banding for morbid obesity: high long-term complication and failure rates. Obes Surg 2006;16(7): 829–35.

[32] O'Brien PE, Dixon JB, Laurie C, et al. A prospective randomized trial of placement of the laparoscopic adjustable gastric band: comparison of the perigastric and pars flaccida pathways. Obes Surg 2005;15(6):820–6.

[33] Westling A, Bjurling K, Ohrvall M, et al. Silicone-adjustable gastric banding: disappointing results. Obes Surg 1998;8(4):467–74.

[34] Silecchia G, Restuccia A, Elmore U, et al. Laparoscopic adjustable silicone gastric banding: prospective evaluation of intragastric migration of the lap-band. Surg Laparosc Endosc Percutan Tech 2001;11(4):229–34.

[35] Camerini G, Adami G, Marinari GM, et al. Thirteen years of follow-up in patients with adjustable silicone gastric banding for obesity: weight loss and constant rate of late specific complications. Obes Surg 2004;14(10):1343–8.

[36] Parikh MS, Fielding GA, Ren CJ. U.S. experience with 749 laparoscopic adjustable gastric bands: intermediate outcomes. Surg Endosc 2005;19(12):1631–5.

[37] DeMaria EJ, Sugerman HJ, Meador JG, et al. High failure rate after laparoscopic adjustable silicone gastric banding for treatment of morbid obesity. Ann Surg 2001;233(6):809–18.

[38] Mason EE, Ito C. Gastric bypass in obesity. Surg Clin North Am 1967;47(6):1345–51.

[39] Griffen WO Jr, Bivins BA, Bell RM, et al. Gastric bypass for morbid obesity. World J Surg 1981;5(6):817–22.

[40] Higa KD, Ho T, Boone KB. Internal hernias after laparoscopic Roux-en-Y gastric bypass: incidence, treatment and prevention. Obes Surg 2003;13(3):350–4.

[41] Cho M, Pinto D, Carrodeguas L, et al. Frequency and management of internal hernias after laparoscopic antecolic antegastric Roux-en-Y gastric bypass without division of the small bowel mesentery or closure of mesenteric defects: review of 1400 consecutive cases. Surg Obes Relat Dis 2006;2(2):87–91.

[42] Hwang RF, Swartz DE, Felix EL. Causes of small bowel obstruction after laparoscopic gastric bypass. Surg Endosc 2004;18(11):1631–5.

[43] Frezza EE, Wachtel MS. Laparoscopic re-exploration in mechanical bowel obstruction after laparoscopic gastric bypass for morbid obesity. Minerva Chir 2006;61(3):193–7.

[44] Bloomberg RD, Fleishman A, Nalle JE, et al. Nutritional deficiencies following bariatric surgery: what have we learned? Obes Surg 2005;15(2):145–54.

[45] Brolin RE, Gorman JH, Gorman RC, et al. Are vitamin B12 and folate deficiency clinically important after roux-en-Y gastric bypass? J Gastrointest Surg 1998;2(5):436–42.

[46] Buchwald H, Avidor Y, Braunwald E, et al. Bariatric surgery: a systematic review and meta-analysis. JAMA 2004;292(14):1724–37.

[47] Hess DS, Hess DW, Oakley RS. The biliopancreatic diversion with the duodenal switch: results beyond 10 years. Obes Surg 2005;15(3):408–16.

[48] Dolan K, Hatzifotis M, Newbury L, et al. A clinical and nutritional comparison of biliopancreatic diversion with and without duodenal switch. Ann Surg 2004;240(1):51–6.

[49] Rabkin RA, Rabkin JM, Metcalf B, et al. Nutritional markers following duodenal switch for morbid obesity. Obes Surg 2004;14(1):84–90.

[50] Ren CJ, Patterson E, Gagner M. Early results of laparoscopic biliopancreatic diversion with duodenal switch: a case series of 40 consecutive patients. Obes Surg 2000;10(6):514–23 [discussion: 24].

[51] Fazylov RM, Savel RH, Horovitz JH, et al. Association of super-super-obesity and male gender with elevated mortality in patients undergoing the duodenal switch procedure. Obes Surg 2005;15(5):618–23.

[52] Almogy G, Crookes PF, Anthone GJ. Longitudinal gastrectomy as a treatment for the high-risk super-obese patient. Obes Surg 2004;14(4):492–7.

[53] Regan JP, Inabnet WB, Gagner M, et al. Early experience with two-stage laparoscopic Roux-en-Y gastric bypass as an alternative in the super-super obese patient. Obes Surg 2003;13(6):861–4.

[54] Cottam D, Qureshi FG, Mattar SG, et al. Laparoscopic sleeve gastrectomy as an initial weight-loss procedure for high-risk patients with morbid obesity. Surg Endosc 2006;20(6):859–63.

[55] Luft HS, Bunker JP, Enthoven AC. Should operations be regionalized? The empirical relation between surgical volume and mortality. N Engl J Med 1979;301(25):1364–9.

[56] Luft HS. The relation between surgical volume and mortality: an exploration of causal factors and alternative models. Med Care 1980;18(9):940–59.

[57] Flood AB, Scott WR, Ewy W. Does practice make perfect? Part I: the relation between hospital volume and outcomes for selected diagnostic categories. Med Care 1984;22(2):98–114.

[58] Sosa JA, Bowman HM, Gordon TA, et al. Importance of hospital volume in the overall management of pancreatic cancer. Ann Surg 1998;228(3):429–38.

[59] Dardik A, Burleyson GP, Bowman H, et al. Surgical repair of ruptured abdominal aortic aneurysms in the state of Maryland: factors influencing outcome among 527 recent cases. J Vasc Surg 1998;28(3):413–20 [discussion: 20–1].

[60] Dardik A, Lin JW, Gordon TA, et al. Results of elective abdominal aortic aneurysm repair in the 1990s: a population-based analysis of 2335 cases. J Vasc Surg 1999;30(6):985–95.

[61] Hannan EL, Popp AJ, Tranmer B, et al. Relationship between provider volume and mortality for carotid endarterectomies in New York state. Stroke 1998;29(11):2292–7.

[62] Harmon JW, Tang DG, Gordon TA, et al. Hospital volume can serve as a surrogate for surgeon volume for achieving excellent outcomes in colorectal resection. Ann Surg 1999;230(3):404–11 [discussion: 11–3].

[63] Katz JN, Losina E, Barrett J, et al. Association between hospital and surgeon procedure volume and outcomes of total hip replacement in the United States Medicare population. J Bone Joint Surg Am 2001;83-A(11):1622–9.

[64] Begg CB, Riedel ER, Bach PB, et al. Variations in morbidity after radical prostatectomy. N Engl J Med 2002;346(15):1138–44.

[65] Hannan EL, Wu C, Ryan TJ, et al. Do hospitals and surgeons with higher coronary artery bypass graft surgery volumes still have lower risk-adjusted mortality rates? Circulation 2003;108(7):795–801.

[66] Barker FG 2nd, Amin-Hanjani S, Butler WE, et al. In-hospital mortality and morbidity after surgical treatment of unruptured intracranial aneurysms in the United States, 1996–2000: the effect of hospital and surgeon volume. Neurosurgery 2003;52(5):995–1007 [discussion: 9].

[67] Higa KD, Boone KB, Ho T. Complications of the laparoscopic Roux-en-Y gastric bypass: 1,040 patients–what have we learned? Obes Surg 2000;10(6):509–13.

[68] Schauer P, Ikramuddin S, Hamad G, et al. The learning curve for laparoscopic Roux-en-Y gastric bypass is 100 cases. Surg Endosc 2003;17(2):212–5.

[69] Courcoulas A, Schuchert M, Gatti G, et al. The relationship of surgeon and hospital volume to outcome after gastric bypass surgery in Pennsylvania: a 3-year summary. Surgery 2003; 134(4):613–21 [discussion: 21–3].

[70] Nguyen NT, Paya M, Stevens CM, et al. The relationship between hospital volume and outcome in bariatric surgery at academic medical centers. Ann Surg 2004;240(4):586–93 [discussion: 93–4].

[71] Dimick JB, Pronovost PJ, Cowan JA, et al. Complications and costs after high-risk surgery: where should we focus quality improvement initiatives? J Am Coll Surg 2003;196(5):671–8.

[72] American College of Surgeons Bariatric Surgery Center Network Levels of Accreditation. ACS, 2006. Available at: http://www.facs.org/cqi/bscn/levelsdefined.html Accessed December 7, 2006.

[73] Rendon SE, Pories WJ. Quality assurance in bariatric surgery. Surg Clin North Am 2005; 85(4):757–71, vi–vii.

ELSEVIER
SAUNDERS

THE MEDICAL
CLINICS
OF NORTH AMERICA

Med Clin N Am 91 (2007) 383–392

Management of the Challenging Bariatric Surgical Patient

Kent R. Van Sickle, MD

*Division of General and Laparoendoscopic Surgery, University of Texas Health Science
Center San Antonio, 7703 Floyd Curl Dr., Mail Code 7842, San Antonio,
TX 78229-3900, USA*

The increase in bariatric operations has been coupled with an increase in new challenges for the primary care physician, particularly in addressing postoperative problems associated with this complex patient population [Table 1]. With the widespread acceptance of both the Roux-en-Y gastric bypass (RYGBP) and the laparoscopic adjustable gastric band (LAGB), more physicians are now seeing an increasing number of challenging patients, including adolescents, the elderly, and the super obese. Also, increasing numbers of reproductive-age women are undergoing weight loss surgery, thus creating unique metabolic and nutritional issues in this subset of patients. The focus of this chapter is centered on familiarizing the primary care physician with important considerations with regard to this specific subgroup of bariatric surgery patients.

Adolescents

In children, the ratio of weight to height changes with growth, thus, body mass index (BMI) criteria for adolescent obesity are calculated using BMI growth charts developed for children by the US Centers for Diseased Control and Prevention. The definition of obesity for children is 95th percentile or more of BMI for age, and children between the 85th and 95th percentile for age are considered overweight [1,2]. Recent estimates have determined the prevalence of obesity in children aged 6 to 11 years has doubled, and the prevalence of obese adolescents aged 12 to 17 years has tripled between 1980 and 2000 [3–5]. Inge and colleagues [5] have recently published a comprehensive review of the comorbidities related to adolescent obesity, and

E-mail address: sickle@uthscsa.edu

medical.theclinics.com

Table 1
Summary of data regarding challenging bariatric patients

Category	Author/year	N	Mean age	Range	Procedure(s) performed	Follow-up	Preoperative BMI	EWL (%)	Morbidity (%)	Mortality (%)
Adolescent										
	Strauss et al., 2001 [42]	17		15-17	RYGBP	up to 8 y	52.4	59		
	Sugerman et al., 2003 [12]	33	16 ± 1	12.4-17.9	30 RYGBP; 3VBNG	up to 14 y	52 ± 11	59		2 (6)
	Widhalm et al., 2004 [10]	8	16 ± 1	15-18	LAGB	1 y	49.1 ± 52	16	n/1	n/1
	Dolan et al., 2003 [8]	17	17[a]	12-19	LAGB	2 y	44.7[a]	58.40	2. (11)	0
	Capella et al., 2003	19		13-9	VBG; RYGBP	up to 10 y	49	n/a		
	Abu-Abeid et al., 2003 [43]	11		11-17	LAGB	6-36 m	46.4	n/a		

Super Obese									
Skull, 2004 [21]	76	39	19–51	LAGB	5 y	69 ± 6.2	46.7 ± 10	n/l	0
Moose et al., 2003 [36]	67	42	19–62	LBP	1 y	57	55	6 (10%)	1 (1.5)
Mongol, 2005 [38]	290	n/a	n/a	LGBP; LAGB	2 y		LGBP, 63 LAGB, 41	LGBP 10 - 26% LAGB - 3–15%	1 (1)
Bloomston et al., 1997 [44]	78	n/a	n/a	VGB; RYGBP	3 y	61	42		1 (1)
Dresel, 2004 [45]	60	40	19–60	LGBP	n/a	58.4	n/a	8–12%	
Tichansky et al., 2005 [39]	45	41.6	n/a	LGBP	1 y	65.6 ± 5.3	58 ± 13	14 (31)	
Cottam, 2006 [34]	126	49.5	20–74	LSG	1 y	65.4 ± 9	45 ± 17	18 (14)	
Silecchia et al., 2006 [46]	41	44		LSG	1 y	57.3			
Elderly									
Sugerman et al., 2004 [12]	80	63 ± 3	n/a	RYGBP	5 y	49 ± 7	57		
Papasavas et al., 2004 [47]	71	59	55–67	LRYGBP	17 mo	50.2	64	22 (32)	1 (1.5)

Abbreviations: LSG, laparoscopic sleeva gastrectomy; n/a, not available; n/l, not listed; VBG, vertical banded gastroplasty.
[a] Median.

other authors have identified significant psychological and social impacts of obesity in children [6].

In July 2004, a panel of experts in adolescent obesity outlined eligibility criteria in patients for whom weight loss surgery is to be considered [7]:

1. Presence of severe obesity (BMI $\geq$ 40).
2. Presence of comorbidities.
3. Skeletal/physiologic maturity.
4. Failure of $\geq$ 6 months of structured attempts at weight loss.
5. Commitment to multidisciplinary evaluations before and after surgery.
6. Commitment and ability to follow nutritional guidelines after surgery.
7. Commitment to avoid pregnancy for $\geq$ 1 year postoperatively.
8. Informed consent.
9. Decision-making capacity.

These guidelines, coupled with the rise in popularity of laparoscopy and proven benefits of the RYGBP in adults, has spurred a recent increase in weight loss surgeries (WLS) for obese adolescents. Currently, a small number of comprehensive adolescent bariatric programs exist in the United States and current recommendations from the American Academy of Pediatrics limit WLS to these types of bariatric centers.

Despite the rapid increase in the number of obese adolescents and the associated comorbidities, the number of WLS performed in this age group has remained quite small. Moreover, published experience of bariatric surgery in adolescence is scant and has limited follow-up [1], and before 2005 an estimate of adolescent WLS in the United States numbered in the hundreds compared with the nearly 200,000 WLS performed in adults annually.

The laparoscopic Roux-en-Y gastric bypass (LRYGBP) currently is considered to be the "gold standard" for WLS in adults and has likewise gained approval for obese adolescents. The LAP-BAND was approved by the Food and Drug Administration in 2001 for adults but is not yet approved in the United States for patients less than 18 years of age. Also, very few (if any) insurance companies pay for the use of this device. Fielding and colleagues have reported their experience with LAGB in Australia [8,9], and Widhalm and colleagues [10] reported early success with the LAP-BAND in Europe. Currently, no U.S. data on adolescents exits with this procedure.

Inge and colleagues [11], has recently reported the early outcomes from their initial experience with LRYGBP in adolescents, and the results are similar to that which has been shown in the adult population, but long-term follow-up and complication rates remain unknown. The largest series with long-term follow-up was reported by Sugerman and colleagues [12] in 2003, which showed effective durable weight loss and resolution of comorbidities in most patients. There were 4 patient deaths found in follow-up but were not believed to be related to the WLS. The most common postoperative complications seen in this series were bowel obstruction, incisional hernias, and weight regain (seen in 15%). Postoperative concerns related to the RYGBP in adolescents mirror those in the adult population and should be addressed in a similar manner.

Pregnancy

Because women of childbearing age represent the largest cohort of patients undergoing weight loss surgery, issues related to WLS and pregnancy are likely to become substantially more common. The effects of bariatric surgery on this cohort can be stratified into two categories: preconception (including contraception) and pregnancy related.

Preconception

Oral contraceptives will have altered absorption from the gut in any patient having undergone gastric bypass and thus may have insufficient levels in the blood to prevent subsequent pregnancy [13]. Subsequently, other routes of administration such as transdermal patches, intramuscular injections, or subcutaneous implants (ie, Norplant) should be recommended. Such recommendations would not be required for women having undergone LAGB, because this is a purely restrictive procedure and will have no impact on the absorption of the contraceptive agent.

The primary concern with regard to WLS and pregnancy is that of nutritional and metabolic consequences. Anemia is by far the most common micronutrient deficiency and can occur in up to two thirds of patients [14], resulting from iron, folate, or vitamin B12 deficiencies. Menstruating women who have undergone gastric bypass are particularly at high risk for iron deficiency anemia [15] because of poor dietary intake, reduced absorption, and decreased exposure to gastric acid. Subsequently, all reproductive-age women should be placed on lifelong oral iron supplements after gastric bypass.

Likewise, deficiencies in B12 and folate have been reported in 70% and 40% of patients undergoing gastric bypass surgery and "downstream" effects of these deficiencies on pregnancy have been reported. An association has been shown between recurrent early pregnancy loss and elevated serum homocysteine levels related to vitamin B deficiency [16]. A case report of an exclusively breast-fed infant developing B12 deficiency, failure to thrive, and megaloblastic anemia also has been described [17].

The cause and effect relationship between folate deficiency and neural tube defects in the newborn has been extensively studied [18–20]. Fortunately, both of these nutrient deficiencies can be easily prevented by daily oral supplementation of vitamin B12 and folate. The easiest and most popular supplements are daily multivitamins, which provide sufficient folic acid and one of either intramuscular preparations or nasal spray administration of vitamin B12.

Pregnancy related

Maternal obesity is a well-recognized risk factor for gestational diabetes and maternal hypertension and is more likely to result in instrumental delivery or caesarean section [21]. Skull and colleagues [21] conducted an observational study of their patients undergoing LAGB during pregnancy and found no adverse outcomes related to the LAP-BAND with an improvement in maternal obesity-related diseases. Likewise, the babies of pregnant LAP-BAND patients had no differences in fetal weight or neonatal complications.

Early case reports and series have described various pregnancy-related complications after bariatric surgery including gastrointestinal bleeding [22], anemia [23], intrauterine growth restriction [24], and neural tube defects [25]. However, these reports do not reflect current standards of therapy (ie, LYRGBP or LAGB), and thus the incidence is exceedingly rare.

Recent studies have found that bariatric surgery is not associated with adverse perinatal outcomes [26]. In fact, some series have shown that pregnancies after WLS are less likely to be complicated by gestational diabetes, hypertension, and macrosomia than pregnancies of obese women who have not had the surgery [18,20,26]. In the study by Sheiner and colleagues [26], the incidence of cesarean delivery was significantly higher in women having undergone WLS (either open or laparoscopic), and thus these patients should be counseled accordingly.

In 2005, two case reports were published showing significant complications of RYGBP related to pregnancy. The first report described intestinal ischemia from a strangulated small bowel obstruction at the site of the Roux limb anastomosis in a 23-year-old woman at 25 weeks' gestation [27] that resulted in fetal demise despite successful operative treatment of the mother. The second report was a series of two patients who presented with small bowel obstruction at differing stages of pregnancy (12 and 34 weeks' gestation, respectively), both of which required laparotomy for treatment but had no adverse effects on the fetus [28].

Fortunately, despite these limited series and case reports, WLS generally has a positive effect on pregnancy particularly in reducing the likelihood of obesity-related complications, such as gestational diabetes, macrosomia, and preeclampsia [29]. Likewise, a woman's fertility improves because of the loss of excess weight and thus it is likely that more physicians will be seeing pregnancies in WLS patients.

Most physicians should advise patients who have undergone WLS that a weight-stable plateau should be achieved before attempting to become pregnant, because this will minimize the nutritional consequences on the fetus. Also, all reproductive-age women should be on daily iron supplements and a multivitamin (for folate) and supplemental vitamin B12 if they have a clinically significant anemia.

Elderly

The rise in popularity of obesity surgery has not been limited to younger patients. A recent article evaluating the trends in bariatric surgery in the United States found a dramatic increase in the number of weight loss procedures in patients age 50 to 64 (15% to 24%) over the last 5 years. However, "elderly" defined in terms of bariatric surgery applies to patients aged 65 and over, and the article by Santry and colleagues [30] found that the number of bariatric procedures in this cohort has remained fairly constant over the last 5 years.

It is well known that morbidity and mortality increase with advancing age, and bariatric surgery is no exception. In a recent landmark article in JAMA, patients age 65 and older were at a significantly higher risk of death (both early and late) after WLS than their younger counterparts [31]. This finding increased the scrutiny surrounding bariatric surgery in the elderly, and now Medicare will not reimburse hospitals for WLS on these patients unless they are performed in so-called "Centers of Excellence" (ie, high-volume hospitals). Subsequently, other insurance companies have followed suit, and, thus, WLS on the elderly has generally been restricted to these tertiary referral centers.

One of the issues surrounding bariatric surgery in the elderly is that traditionally most patients age 65 and over were deliberately excluded from clinical trials involving weight loss (medical or surgical). Given the findings from Flum and colleagues [31], that scenario is unlikely to change. However, it has been demonstrated in many recent studies that both gastric bypass and the LAP-BAND are safe and efficacious in elderly patients [32,33]. The effects of WLS in this cohort are similar to that of younger patients and the resolution of comorbidities is equally dramatic and significant. Currently, elderly patients whose life expectancy is 5 years or greater are evaluated similarly to younger patients. Although advanced age is not a contraindication for a weight loss procedure, the current recommendations are for these high-risk patients to be evaluated and treated in an established bariatric Center of Excellence, because the data have shown that complication rates are lower in this age group than in low-volume centers.

Super obese

Super obese patients are defined as those with a BMI ≥ 50 kg/m^2. Traditionally, complications from WLS are much higher in this subgroup of patients [34–37], and, as a result, many bariatric programs do not offer WLS to patients with BMIs in this range. However, refinements in surgical technique and improvements with laparoscopic equipment have facilitated the safety and feasibility of performing WLS in this group. Several investigators have recently reported their success with either the LAP-BAND or the laparoscopic RYGBP (or both) in the super obese [36,38–40]. Complication rates in these patients do not appear to be significantly different from those with BMIs <50 kg/m^2, and the weight loss results are similar.

Limited evidence exists as to whether the LAP-BAND or the LRYGBP is the better weight loss procedure for the super obese. A retrospective study by Mognol and colleagues [38] compared complication rates and weight loss in super obese patients undergoing either LAP-BAND or LRYGBP and found that although initial weight loss was better in the LRYGBP group, complication rates were higher. Because of the lack of convincing data, some investigators have advocated a two-stage approach for super obese patients [37,41]. The concept of a two-stage approach is to perform a gastric-restrictive procedure initially (either a partial or so-called "sleeve" gastrectomy or a gastric banding), that is then followed by a malabsorptive procedure (either gastric bypass or a duodenal switch) once the weight loss from the initial procedure has reached its plateau.

A recent study published by Cottam and colleagues [34] showed that a two-stage approach can be done safely using laparoscopic sleeve gastrectomy as the initial weight loss procedure followed by a LRYGBP. Because both approaches were able to be performed laparoscopically, and the current gold standard (ie, LRYGBP) was used as the second procedure, this approach is likely to become more of an attractive option in the super obese patient. However, because this approach involves two operations and requires close follow-up in a high-risk patient population, the two-stage concept has not yet been adopted as the standard of care for this cohort. Also, refinements of both the LAP-BAND and LRYGBP have made either of these approaches an accepted treatment in most super obese individuals.

Summary

Despite the continued increase in surgical procedures for weight loss, the dramatic increase in the prevalence of morbid obesity far outpaces the treatments to correct it. As a result, the primary care physician is increasingly more likely to be evaluating patients who are either candidates for weight loss surgery or who have already undergone a weight loss procedure. Unique medical and social situations must be considered when evaluating these patients, and it is anticipated that all physicians will be seeing a greater number of complex or challenging patients. Extremes in age are not a contraindication for weight loss surgery but need to be evaluated within the context of a comprehensive weight management program. Women of childbearing age represent the largest cohort of weight loss surgery patients, and the nutritional and metabolic consequences of WLS need to be addressed before conception if possible. Super obese patients are no longer considered to be too "high risk," although the ideal weight loss procedure has not been established for this group.

References

[1] Garcia VF, Langford L, Inge TH. Application of laparoscopy for bariatric surgery in adolescents. Curr Opin Pediatr 2003;15:248–55.

[2] Helmrath MA, Brandt ML, Inge TH. Adolescent obesity and bariatric surgery. Surg Clin North Am 2006;86:441–554.

[3] Apovian CM, Baker C, Ludwig DS, et al. Best practice guidelines in pediatric/adolescent weight loss surgery. Obes Res 2005;13(2):274–82.

[4] Rodgers BM. Bariatric surgery for adolescents: a view from the American Pediatric Surgical Association. Pediatrics 2004;114:255–6.

[5] Inge TH, Krebs NF, Garcia VF, et al. Bariatric surgery for severely overweight adolescents: concerns and recommendations. Pediatrics 2004;114(1):217–23.

[6] Zeller MG, Roehrig HR, Modi AC, et al. Health-related quality of life and depressive symptoms in adolescents with extreme obesity presenting for bariatric surgery. Pediatrics 2006; 117(4):1155–61.

[7] Durant N, Cox J. Current treatment approaches to overweight in adolescents. Curr Opin Pediatr 2005;17(4):454–9.

[8] Dolan K, Creighton L, Hopkins G, et al. Laparoscopic gastric banding in morbidly obese adolescents. Obes Surg 2003;13(1):101–4.

[9] Fielding GA, Duncombe JE. Laparoscopic adjustable gastric banding in severely obese adolescents. Surg Obes Relat Dis 2005;1(4):399–405 [discussion: 405–7].

[10] Widhalm K, Dietrich S, Prager G. Adjustable gastric banding surgery in morbidly obese adolescents: experiences with eight patients. Int J Obes 2004;28:S42–5.

[11] Inge TH, Garcia V, Daniels S, et al. A multidisciplinary approach to the adolescent bariatric surgical patient. J Pediatr Surg 2004;39(3):442–7 [discussion: 446–7].

[12] Sugerman HJ, Sugerman EL, DeMaria EJ, et al. Bariatric surgery for severely obese adolescents. J Gastrointest Surg 2003;7(1):102–8.

[13] Deitel M. Pregnancy after bariatric surgery. Obes Surg 1998;8:465–6.

[14] Xanthakos SA, Inge TH. Nutritional consequences of bariatric surgery. Curr Opin Clin Nutr Metab Care 2006;9(4):489–96.

[15] Lynch RJ, Eisenberg D, Bell RL. Metabolic consequences of bariatric surgery. J Clin Gastroenterol 2006;40(8):659–68.

[16] Nelen WL, Blom HJ, Steegers EA, et al. Homocysteine and folate levels as risk factors for recurrent early pregnancy loss. Obstetrics & Gynecology 2000;95(4):519–24.

[17] Grange DK, Finlay JL. Nutritional vitamin B12 deficiency in a breastfed infant following maternal gastric bypass. Pediatr Hematol Oncol 1994;11(3):311–8.

[18] Martin L, Finigan K, Nolan TE. Pregnancy after adjustable gastric banding. Obstetrics & Gynecology 2000;95:927–30.

[19] Weiss HG, Nehoda H, Labeck B, et al. Pregnancies after adjustable gastric banding. Obes Surg 2001;11:303–6.

[20] Wittgrove AC, Jester L, Wittgrove P, et al. Pregnancy following gastric bypass for morbid obesity. Obes Surg 1998;8:461–4 [discussion: 465–6].

[21] Skull AJ, Slater GH, Duncombe JE, et al. Laparoscopic adjustable banding in pregnancy: safety, patient tolerance and effect on obesity-related pregnancy outcomes. Obes Surg 2004;14(2):230–5.

[22] Ramirez MM, Turrentine MA. Gastrointestinal hemorrhage during pregnancy in a patient with a history of vertical-banded gastroplasty. Am J Obstet Gynecol 1995;173(5):1630–1.

[23] Gurewitsch ED, Smith-Levitin M, Mack J. Pregnancy following gastric bypass surgery for morbid obesity. Obstetrics & Gynecology 1996;88(4 Pt 2):658–61.

[24] Granstrom L, Granstrom L, Backman L. Fetal growth retardation after gastric banding. Acta Obstet Gynecol Scand 1990;69(6):533–6.

[25] Haddow JE, Hill LE, Kloza EM, et al. Neural tube defects after gastric bypass. Lancet 1986; 1:1330.

[26] Sheiner E, Levy A, Silverberg D, et al. Pregnancy after bariatric surgery is not associated with adverse perinatal outcome. Am J Obstet Gynecol 2004;190:1335–40.

[27] Charles A, Domingo S, Goldfadden A, et al. Small bowel ischemia after Roux-en-Y gastric bypass complicated by pregnancy: a case report. Am Surg 2005;71:231–4.

[28] Kakarla N, Dailey C, Marino T, et al. Pregnancy after gastric bypass surgery and internal hernia formation. Obstet Gynecol 2005;105(NO. 5 Part 2):1195–8.

[29] Woodard CB. Pregnancy following bariatric surgery. J Perinat Neonatal Nurs 2004;18(4): 329–40.

[30] Santry HP, Gillen DL, Lauderdale DS. Trends in bariatric surgical procedures. JAMA 2005;294(15):1909–17.

[31] Flum DR, Salem L, Elrod JA, et al. Early mortality among Medicare beneficiaries undergoing bariatric surgical procedures. JAMA 2005;294:1903–8.

[32] Varela J, Wilson SE, Nguyen N. Outcomes of bariatric surgery in the elderly. American Surgeon 2006;72(10):865–9.

[33] Sugerman HJ, DeMaria EJ, Kellum JM, et al. Effects of bariatric surgery in older patients. Annals of Surgery 2004;240(2):24–7.

[34] Cottam D, Qureshi FG, Mattar SG, et al. Laparoscopic sleeve gastrectomy as an initial weight-loss procedure for high-risk patients with morbid obesity. Surg Endosc 2006;20: 859–63.

[35] Fielding GA. Laparoscopic adjustable gastric banding for massive superobesity (> 60 body mass index kg/m^2). Surg Endosc 2003;17(10):1541–5.

[36] Moose D, Lourie D, Powell W, et al. Laparoscopic Roux-en-Y gastric bypass: minimally invasive bariatric surgery for the superobese in the community hospital setting. Am Surg 2003; 69:930–2.

[37] Regan JP, Inabnet WB, Gagner M, et al. Early experience with two-stage laparoscopic Roux-en-Y gastric bypass as an alternative in the super-super obese patient. Obes Surg 2003;13(6):861–4.

[38] Mognol P, Chosidow D, Marmuse JP. Laparoscopic gastric bypass versus laparoscopic adjustable gastric banding in the super-obese: a comparative study of 290 patients. Obes Surg 2005;15(1):76–8196.

[39] Tichansky DS, DeMaria EJ, Fernandez AZ, et al. Postoperative complications are not increased in super-obese patients who undergo laparoscopic Roux-en-Y gastric bypass. Surgical Endoscopy 2005;19(7):939–41.

[40] Parikh MS, Fielding GA, Ren CJ. U.S. experience with 749 laparoscopic adjustable gastric bands. Surg Endosc 2005;19:1631–5.

[41] Chu CA, Gagner M, Quinn T, et al. Two-stage laparoscopic biliopancreatic diversion with duodenal switch: an alternative approach to super-super morbid obesity. Surg Endosc 2002; 16:S187.

[42] Strauss RS, Brolin RE. Gastric bypass surgery in adolescents with morbid obesity. Journal of Pediatrics 2001;138:499–504.

[43] Abu-Abeid S, Gavert N, Klausner J. Bariatric surgery in adolescence. Journal of Pediatric Surgery 2003;38(9):1379–82.

[44] Bloomston M, Zervos E, Camps M. Outcome following bariatric surgery in super versus morbid obese patients: does weight matter? Obesity Surgery 1997;7(5):414–9.

[45] Dresel A, Kuhn JA, McCarty TM. Laparoscopic Roux-en-Y gastric bypass in morbidly obese and super morbidly obese patients. American Journal of Surgery 2004;187(2):230–2.

[46] Silecchia G, Boru C, Pecchia A. Effectiveness of laparoscopic sleeve gastrectomy (first stage of biliopancreatic diversion with duodenal switch) on co-morbidities in super-obese high-risk patients. Obesity Surgery 2006;16(9):1138–44.

[47] Papasavas PK, Gagner DJ, Kelly J, et al. Laparoscopic Roux-en-Y gastric bypass is a safe and effective operation for the treatment of morbid obesity in patients older than 55 years. Obesity Surgery 2004;14(8):1056–61.

ELSEVIER
SAUNDERS

THE MEDICAL
CLINICS
OF NORTH AMERICA

Med Clin N Am 91 (2007) 393–414

Metabolic Aspects of Bariatric Surgery

Franco Folli, MD, Phd[a],*, Antonio E. Pontiroli, MD[b],
Wayne H. Schwesinger, MD[c],*

[a]Department of Medicine, Diabetes Division, University of Texas Health Science Center,
7703 Floyd Curl Drive, San Antonio, TX 78229, USA
[b]Department of Medicine, University of Milano, Ospedale San Paolo,
Via Di Rudini, 20100 Milano, Italy
[c]Department of Surgery, University of Texas Health Science Center,
7703 Floyd Curl Drive, San Antonio, TX 78229, USA

The metabolic consequences of obesity are well known but incompletely understood. They include insulin resistance, type 2 diabetes mellitus (T2DM), the metabolic syndrome, and polycystic ovary syndrome (PCOS). Each disorder develops as a result of the poorly defined interaction between a genetic predisposition and other acquired and environmental factors such as age, gender, ethnicity, dietary choices, and level of physical activity. Taken together, these disorders have become an increasing source of morbidity worldwide as the obesity pandemic continues to spread. It is generally agreed that the global prevalence of insulin resistance is continuing to increase. In the United States, diabetes is the sixth leading cause of death and continues to be a major cause of blindness, renal failure, peripheral neuropathy, and amputation [1]. It is now estimated that 90% of all diabetes cases are T2DM [2]. The economic cost is already enormous and growing. In 2002, T2DM was responsible for at least $132 billion in medical expenditures and lost productivity [3]. By 2020, the overall cost is projected to reach a staggering $192 billion annually.

It is well documented that the metabolic problems associated with obesity can be partially or completely reversed, but only with early and aggressive therapy. Accordingly, a variety of medical and surgical treatments are now available and new ones continue to evolve. The time-honored approaches of diet, exercise, and behavioral modification can achieve a 10% to 15% reduction in body weight and significantly enhance insulin sensitivity and glycemic control in the short term [4]. Nonetheless, the extended

* Corresponding authors.
E-mail addresses: folli@uthscsa.edu (F. Folli); schwesinger@uthscsa.edu (W.H. Schwesinger).

results of nonoperative therapy continue to be disappointing because protracted compliance is difficult and weight loss tends to be unsustainable [5].

An important role for surgery in the management of these difficult problems was first suggested over a decade ago by the breakthrough work of Pories and colleagues [6] in which a rapid and durable resolution of T2DM was observed following gastric bypass operations. Since then, numerous other investigators have confirmed and extended these findings using a wide range of bariatric procedures. This cumulative experience has helped to promote a dramatic growth in the volume of bariatric surgery. In addition, it has stimulated multidisciplinary efforts to better understand the pathophysiology of obesity-specific metabolic diseases and to determine the most appropriate therapeutic targets. Some of the results are discussed herein.

Insulin resistance

Insulin is a potent anabolic/pleiotropic hormone that is primarily responsible for glucose homeostasis but is also involved in fat and protein metabolism, endothelial nitric oxide synthesis, and cell differentiation and growth. It acts to maintain plasma glucose within a reasonably narrow range by a complex interaction primarily with insulin-sensitive cells of the liver, adipose tissue, and skeletal muscle. At a cellular level, insulin promotes the transport of glucose from the bloodstream into the cytoplasm by binding to a specific surface receptor and initiating an intracytoplasmic, multistep signaling pathway that leads to activation of glucose transporter 4 (GLUT4). This pathway involves phosphorylation of intracellular receptor substrates (proteins), which, in turn, activate several additional pathways, the most important of which is the PI-3 kinase/PDK-1-AKT pathway [7]. In vivo, the main effects of insulin on glucose metabolism are to suppress hepatic glucose production by inhibiting hepatic gluconeogenesis and glycogen breakdown and to promote the transport of glucose from the bloodstream into peripheral tissues, especially skeletal muscle.

Insulin resistance is defined as the inability of insulin to produce its usual biologic effects at circulating concentrations that are otherwise effective in normal subjects. It is the central metabolic abnormality associated with obesity and is present in the great majority of morbidly obese patients. In obese diabetic and nondiabetic subjects and in animal models, there is a reduction of insulin receptor number as well as decreased insulin receptor phosphorylation, IRS-1 and IRS-2 phosphorylation, and activation of PI-3 kinase. It is likely that other factors are affected as well [8,9].

Insulin resistance is heterogeneous in its expression. It is associated with impaired suppression of glucose output by the liver and reduced postprandial uptake of glucose, primarily by muscle. In addition, it is accompanied by increased triglyceride breakdown in adipose tissue with generation of free fatty acids, which further interferes with insulin action and glucose metabolism. The specific pathogenesis of these molecular defects in humans is not yet clearly defined but important clues are beginning to emerge; all point to the participation of multiple factors (Fig. 1) [10].

The most common but still elusive factor is a genetic predisposition. In this regard, polymorphisms of certain genes (*IRS-1, IL-6, PPrγ, PC-1, UCP-2*) have previously been demonstrated to predispose to insulin resistance and T2DM in selected ethnic groups [11,12]. Furthermore, epidemiologic studies of affected twins, first-degree relatives, and American Indians suggest the importance of genetic factors [13,14].

Advanced age can also promote insulin resistance. This effect is explained in part by the changes in body composition that occur with aging, such as losses in muscle mass and gains in total and visceral fat content [15]. In addition, the reduction in physical activity that typically accompanies aging is a major independent risk factor for insulin resistance at whatever age [16,17]. At a subcellular level, the reduced ATP synthesis that occurs as

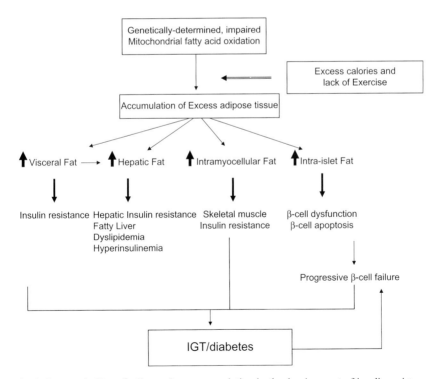

Fig. 1. Proposed effect of adipose tissue accumulation in the development of insulin resistance and type 2 diabetes. (*From* Rattarasarn C. Physiological and pathophysiological regulation of regional adipose tissue in the development of insulin resistance and type 2 diabetes. Acta Physiologica 2006;186:87–101).

a result of age-related mitochondrial degradation has been demonstrated to impair insulin function [18].

Obesity is linked to insulin resistance through a variety of injurious cellular events, most of which result from lipid oversupply, so-called "lipotoxicity." In part, this is a manifestation of the chronic accumulation of excess fat within hepatocytes, myocytes, and adipocytes with resultant perturbation of the molecular mechanisms of insulin signaling.

In skeletal muscle, major defects occur in oxidative capacity secondary to elevated levels of long chain acyl CoA and the subsequent activation of protein kinase C isoforms with or without accumulation of ceramide [19,20]. Other unspecified mechanisms are undoubtedly involved. Parenthetically, accumulation of intramyocellular lipids is also observed in endurance athletes but, in this setting, is associated with increased rather than decreased insulin sensitivity. This "metabolic flexibility" is due to an essential shift of energy metabolism from glucose to lipid oxidation [21].

It is well known that excess fat also accumulates in adipose cells and contributes to insulin resistance, but many of the steps in this sequence remain undefined. It is generally accepted that the pattern of fat distribution is an important predictor of risk. Individuals with predominantly upper body fat (visceral/android obesity) are more likely to be insulin resistant and hyperinsulinemic than are people with a preponderance of lower body fat (gynoid obesity). This association of insulin resistance with visceral obesity has been attributed, in part, to the enhanced lipolytic activity of visceral fat cells, especially in the omentum, with increased delivery of free fatty acids into the portal and systemic circulations and chronic exposure of hepatocytes and myocytes to high free fatty acid levels. Several mechanistic studies performed in rodents support the concept that increased free fatty acids have an important role in the pathogenesis of insulin resistance [22].

Chronic, low-grade inflammation in adipose tissue has also been implicated in insulin resistance and has been cited as an important cause of the extraordinary risk of cardiovascular disease observed in patients with obesity and T2DM [23].

Excess fat in adipose cells can induce increased secretion of monocyte chemoattractant protein-1 (MCP-1), which is a mediator for macrophage recruitment. The infiltrating inflammatory cells may, in turn, secrete a variety of chemokines and cytokines (eg, interleukin-6 [IL-6], interferon–γ) that further promote the local inflammatory response and secondarily affect gene expression in adipocytes, resulting in systemic insulin resistance [24].

Individual adipocytes are now recognized to have a central role in the pathogenesis of obesity-related insulin resistance. They are highly specialized cells that not only store triglyceride but also serve as a source of various regulatory peptides (adipokines) that can trigger a wide range of metabolic and inflammatory processes. The specific signals that initiate adipokine secretion remain to be completely determined, but the mechanical stress of adipocyte swelling, intracellular oxidative stress, and endoplasmic reticulum stress are well-recognized candidates [25,26].

Adiponectin (Acrp30 or adipoQ) is the most abundant known adipokine and has several unique characteristics. It is expressed only in adipocytes and is secreted directly into the circulation, and it is the only known adipocyte-secreted factor that increases tissue sensitivity to insulin. This increased sensitivity is accomplished, in part, by the promotion of lipid uptake and oxidation in muscle and by the inhibition of triglyceride synthesis in hepatocytes [27]. Accordingly, plasma adiponectin levels are inversely related to visceral obesity, T2DM, hypertension, and coronary artery disease [28,29].

Leptin, another potent adipokine, acts primarily through hypothalamic receptors to regulate food intake and energy homeostasis [30]. It is considered an independent risk factor for cardiovascular diseases and is released in proportion to excess body weight. Significant molecular cross-talk has been demonstrated between leptin- and insulin- signaling networks, especially in the liver, but no clear relationship to insulin resistance has been established [31,32]. Other insulin-resistant adipokines, such as resistin, retinol-binding protein 4, tumor necrosis factor alpha, IL-6, plasminogen activator inhibitor, and MCP-1, can be increased in obesity but are less well understood [33].

Insulin resistance syndrome

In his 1988 Banting lecture, Reaven [34] first introduced the concept of Syndrome X as a cluster of related physiologic disorders that could predict an increased risk of cardiovascular disease. The specific disorders in his syndrome were insulin resistance, central obesity, hypertriglyceridemia, low high-density lipoprotein (HDL), arterial hypertension, and altered glucose metabolism. Since that initial description, the World Health Organization, the National Cholesterol Education Program Adult Treatment Panel III (NCEP-ATPIII), and the International Diabetes Federation have all modified the original criteria. Nevertheless, in each case, the intent has remained the same, that is, to have a tool that will reliably identify high-risk individuals and prevent the long-term progression of metabolic and cardiovascular disease (Table 1) [35].

The name of the syndrome has been changed several times (insulin resistance syndrome [IRS], metabolic syndrome, dysmetabolic syndrome), and a specific ICD9 code (277.7) has been assigned. Patients affected by the IRS have a twofold increase in the risk of cardiovascular disease and a fivefold increase in the risk of T2DM when compared with unaffected individuals [36].

Ischemic and non-ischemic mechanisms may be involved in the elevated risk of cardiovascular disease. In Sweden, Hulthe and colleagues [37] performed carotid and femoral artery ultrasound studies on 818 asymptomatic,

Table 1
Abnormalities of the insulin resistance syndrome

Parameter	Abnormal value
Triglycerides	> 150 mg/dL
HDL cholesterol	
Men	< 40 mg/dL
Women	< 50 mg/dL
Blood pressure	> 130/85 mm Hg
Glucose	
Fasting	110–125 mg/dL
120-min post glucose challenge	140–200 mg/dL

nondiabetic, 58-year-old men. The IRS was diagnosed in 62 subjects (16%) and was associated with a significant increase in the rate of preclinical atherosclerosis and the presence of a small low-density lipoprotein (LDL) particle size pattern. Depres and colleagues [38] studied patients from the Quebec Cardiovascular Study cohort and noted that fasting hyperinsuline-mia was an independent predictor for ischemic heart disease in nondiabetic men. In another study of 700 subjects undergoing coronary angiography, Saely and colleagues [39] noted that the IRS was an independent predictor of new vascular events within several years. Similarly, studies of coronary artery calcification using electron beam tomography have demonstrated a significant and independent association between such calcification and the IRS and insulin resistance [40]. The mechanisms responsible for the increased risk of atherosclerosis are complex and not firmly established. As summarized by DeFronzo and Ferrannini [41], increased insulin concentrations enhance very low-density lipoprotein (VLDL) synthesis by the liver leading to hypertriglyceridemia. Moreover, elimination of lipid and lipoproteins from the VLDL particle results in the formation of further intermediate- and low-density lipoproteins. All of these processes are atherogenic.

Indirect evidence also indicates that ectopic lipid accumulation in the human myocardium may lead to non-ischemic, functional alterations. In the Strong Heart study of American Indians, an ethnic group known to have a higher prevalence of insulin resistance, impaired glucose tolerance and T2DM were found to be associated with myocardial hypertrophy and systolic and diastolic dysfunction [42]. Similarly, in the Framingham Heart Study, a direct correlation was observed between insulin resistance and echocardiographically determined left ventricular mass, with significant ventricular hypertrophy found in insulin-resistant patients [43]. In a pathologic study, Sharma and colleagues [44] found that intramyocellular lipid overload was present in 30% of non-ischemic failing hearts in biopsy specimens. The excess lipid accumulation was particularly notable in patients with obesity (body mass index [BMI] > 30) and diabetes. Collectively, these and other data suggest that cardiac lipotoxicity is an entity that may contribute to the risk of cardiovascular disease in the IRS.

The therapeutic implications of the IRS are being vigorously debated. Its clinical relevance and utility as a stand-alone syndrome have recently been questioned by its original proponent and by the American Diabetes Association and the European Association for the Study of Diabetes [45,46]. Variations in the philosophical approach to, and the diagnostic criteria of, the three different versions of the IRS have been cited as major concerns. Conversely, the American Association of Clinical Endocrinologists and the American Heart Association have strongly endorsed the IRS concept. Grundy [47] has noted that diagnosis of the IRS imposes a cardiovascular disease risk that is greater than the sum of its parts. He has also suggested that certain metabolic risk factors such as a proinflammatory state and a prothrombotic state, which are not included in standard risk algorithms, become accessible for treatment based on a diagnosis of IRS. Using the recent clinical guidelines proposed by the American Heart Association/ National Heart, Lung, and Blood Institute, the diagnosis of IRS can be conferred by the presence of three or more abnormalities from the following list: central obesity (increased waist circumference), elevated triglycerides, reduced HDL cholesterol, hypertension, and elevated fasting glucose [48].

The therapeutic strategy advocated for patients with multiple risk factors, whether labeled as the IRS or not, is to target the individual risk factors with appropriate medications using available guidelines [49]. The problems associated with polypharmacy, such as poor compliance and adverse drug interactions, require special attention. Lifestyle modification is a critically important but generally underused aspect of therapy. It can reduce medication use, control risk factors, and decrease the long-term risk of cardiovascular disease. In the aggregate, these difficulties suggest a potential role for bariatric surgery [50].

Diabetes mellitus

Diabetes is the prototypical insulin-resistant state. In its earliest phase, muscle, liver, and adipose tissue all become progressively insulin resistant but plasma glucose levels and glucose tolerance remain normal because of a compensatory increase in circulating insulin. Histologically, this phase is associated with hypertrophy and hyperplasia of the beta cells in the pancreatic islets of Langerhans. Over time, impaired glucose tolerance develops and gradually progresses to overt T2DM as beta cells become incapable of increasing their secretion of insulin to compensate for the defect in insulin action (Fig. 2) [51].

In large clinical series, obesity is the single most important predictor of T2DM [52]. The risk of developing T2DM is exponentially related to the BMI, with approximately 40% of morbidly obese patients (BMI > 40) having either impaired fasting glucose or impaired glucose tolerance and nearly 20% developing T2DM [53]. This close association is so prevalent

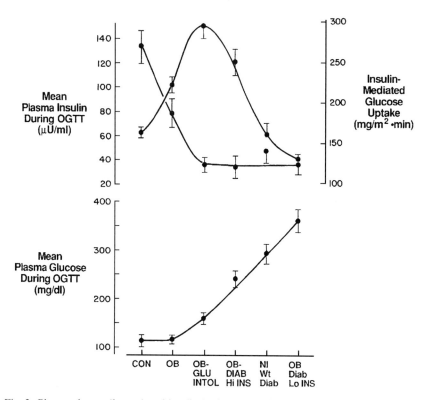

Fig. 2. Plasma glucose (*bottom*) and insulin (*top*) response during 100-g oral glucose tolerance test (OGTT) and tissue sensitivity to insulin (*top*) in control (CON), obese nondiabetic (OB), obese glucose-intolerant (OB-GLU INTOL), obese hyperinsulinemic diabetic (OB-DIAB Hi INS), normal weight diabetic (Nl Wt Diab), and obese hypoinsulinemic diabetic subjects (OB Diab Lo INS). (*From* Defronzo RA. Lilly lecture 1987. The triumvirate: beta-cell, muscle, liver. A collusion responsible for NIDDM. Diabetes 1988;37:667–87. Copyright © 1988 American Diabetes Association; reprinted with permission.)

that it has been termed *diabesity* [54]. It has been documented to affect both genders, all races, and all ages, although the risk is clearly higher in women, non-Hispanic blacks, American Indians/Alaska natives, and Mexican Americans. Particularly alarming is the recent increase in the prevalence of obesity and T2DM in adolescents, especially in minority populations [55]. Overall, diabesity is associated with significant disability, a poorer quality of life, an increased malignancy risk, and premature death. In a follow-up of the first National Health and Nutrition Examination Survey, at least 70% of T2DM patients died of cardiovascular disease [56]. In 2000, the excess global mortality attributable to diabetes was estimated to be 2.9 million deaths or 5.9% of all deaths worldwide [57].

Because of the chronic, progressive, and heterogeneous nature of diabesity, its management is complex and must be long term. If successful, the treatment plan can ameliorate the symptoms of the involved disease processes and control their complications. As described in comprehensive reviews by Scheen [58] and by Campbell and Rossner [59], therapy is based on a multimodal strategy: (1) weight reduction through lifestyle modification together with the selective use of anti-obesity drugs (orlistat, sibutramine); (2) improved blood glucose control with agents from one or more of the following groups: biguanides (metformin), which suppress hepatic glucose production and improve insulin sensitivity; sulfonylureas (glimepiride, glipizide, glyburide, acetohexamide, chlorpropamide), which increase pancreatic insulin secretion; thiazolidinediones (pioglitazone, rosiglitazone), which increase sensitivity to insulin; α-glucosidase inhibitors (acarbose and miglitol), which decrease postprandial hyperglycemia by reducing gastrointestinal carbohydrate absorption; and meglitinides (repaglinide and nateglinide), which increase pancreatic secretion of insulin through a different receptor than that employed by sulfonylureas; and (3) control of common associated risk factors such as arterial hypertension and dyslipidemia.

Although these approaches may be reasonably successful in well-motivated overweight and obese patients, they have little efficacy in the subset of morbid obesity. In large part, this is related to the high rates of recidivism that are observed in nonsurgical weight loss programs [60]. It is also a reflection of the difficulty experienced in medically managing the severe degrees of insulin resistance that are usually present. These challenges provide a strong rationale for the selective use of surgical methods.

Polycystic ovary syndrome

PCOS is a common but complex female endocrinopathy affecting 5% to 10% of women of reproductive age [61]. The primary abnormality is an increase in ovarian androgen production, predominantly testosterone, which results in various combinations of anovulation, menstrual irregularities, infertility, hirsuitism, and acne. The etiology of PCOS is not well understood but appears to be multifactorial, with genetic predisposition being a crucial component. It has reproductive and metabolic phenotypes.

Obesity, especially when visceral in distribution, also appears to be an important etiologic factor, occurring in approximately 30% to 75% of all women with PCOS. Moreover, nearly two thirds of affected individuals are insulin resistant, with the degree of insulin resistance showing a strong positive correlation with the hyperandrogenemia [62]. In this regard, the associated hyperinsulinemia is thought to promote androgen hypersecretion both directly by stimulation of specific ovarian insulin receptors and indirectly by the stimulation of pituitary luteinizing hormone secretion [63].

In addition to the reproductive and cosmetic aspects of PCOS, significant metabolic consequences are increasingly being identified. Notably, impaired glucose tolerance or T2DM has been reported in 40% to 45% of all PCOS patients, with the rate of conversion from normal glucose tolerance to impaired tolerance being significantly increased [64]. Dyslipidemia is also common, with a prevalence of up to 70%. Noninvasive morphologic studies of carotid and coronary arteries have generally demonstrated evidence of early atherosclerosis. Available epidemiologic studies of fatal and nonfatal coronary and cerebrovascular disease have demonstrated at least modest increases in relative risk related to PCOS [65,66]. Definitive conclusions about outcomes will require larger studies with longer follow-up.

The medical and surgical management of PCOS is complex and beyond the scope of this article. Excellent reviews are available [67,68]. Treatment of insulin resistance has become increasingly important. Even a modest level of diet-induced weight loss in obese PCOS patients results in improved insulin sensitivity and lower androgen levels and can ameliorate many of the clinical signs and symptoms of PCOS, including oligomenorrhea, amenorrhea, and anovulation [69]. In patients who are not overweight or who do not respond to diet and exercise, pharmacologic therapy with insulin-sensitizing agents such as metformin (a biguanide) and the thiazolidinediones (pioglitazone and rosiglitazone) is effective and safe. In a recent systematic review, metformin was shown to be better than placebo in achieving ovulation in women with PCOS [70]. In addition, it has been found to correct the associated dyslipidemias and to improve health-related quality of life [71,72].

Surgical management

The role of bariatric surgery in the management of the metabolic problems associated with morbid obesity continues to evolve. The NIH Consensus Development Conference on Gastrointestinal Surgery for Obesity (1991) recognized the importance of certain high-risk comorbid conditions including T2DM and proposed that the BMI threshold for surgical therapy could be dropped from 40 to 35 in appropriate patients [73]. A more recent nongovernmental Consensus Panel co-sponsored by the American Society for Bariatric Surgery (ASBS) and the ASBS Foundation suggested that further liberalization of the operative BMI threshold to 30 may be warranted in the presence of severe comorbidities [74]. This viewpoint has gained increased tenability as minimally invasive techniques have gained more widespread acceptance and as our understanding of the pathobiology of T2DM has improved [75,76]. More randomized clinical studies will be necessary to help determine the need for, and appropriateness of, further changes in the guidelines for bariatric surgical practice [77,78].

The bariatric procedures that are currently available can be divided into three general categories: malabsorptive, restrictive, and combined. Their history and the specific characteristics of each procedure are well discussed in other sources [79,80]. Efficacy and safety profiles differ slightly among the procedural categories, presumably because of the differences in surgical techniques and the variations in physiologic mechanisms.

Malabsorptive techniques induce weight loss by diverting nutrients away from the majority of the small bowel and directly into the distal ileum. Two procedures are now used, biliopancreatic diversion (BPD) and the duodenal switch (DS). For both techniques, general acceptance has been limited because of the relatively frequent side effects of diarrhea, flatulence, anemia, and bone demineralization.

Purely restrictive procedures induce weight loss by combining a small gastric pouch with a narrow outlet, thereby limiting oral intake and producing early satiety. Examples include the vertical banded gastroplasty (VBG), which was used extensively during the 1990s, and its contemporary replacement, the laparoscopic adjustable gastric band (LAGB). The LAGB consists of a water-filled Silastic cuff that is placed around the upper stomach and attached to a subcutaneous port to allow regular adjustments in the size of the gastric outlet.

The Roux-en-Y gastric bypass (RYGB) is the current gold standard of bariatric procedures in the United States and has restrictive and malabsorptive effects. This duality is accomplished by combining a small pouch with a 70- to 150-cm long jejunoileal limb that is excluded from bile and digestive enzymes. Moreover, because nutrients enter directly from the gastric pouch into the jejunum, injudicious carbohydrate intake may cause symptoms of the "dumping syndrome," such as diaphoresis, tachycardia, nausea, and weakness, which provides a strong disincentive for most "sweet-eaters."

To date, most outcome-based studies pertain to T2DM in which the effect is often dramatic and usually rapid, being apparent within days of the operation. This level of improvement cannot be approximated using any currently available nonoperative methods. In the initial Greenville cohort of 608 gastric bypass patients first reported in 1995, a subset of 165 patients was found to have T2DM while another 165 patients demonstrated impaired glucose tolerance. In both groups, it was reported that postoperative glucose metabolism normalized with "surprising speed" [6]. Importantly, during a follow-up period of up to 14 years, euglycemia persisted in 88.5% of the T2DM group and 92.1% of the impaired glucose tolerance group. In a subsequent nonrandomized study from the same center, 154 surgical patients were compared with 78 patients who were managed without operation because of personal preference or insurance difficulties [81]. In the surgical group, the prevalence of T2DM decreased from 31.8% in the pre-study period to 8.6% at the last postoperative follow-up. In the nonoperative group, the prevalence actually increased from 56.4% to 87.5%.

In the largest prospective series reported to date, the Swedish Obese Subjects study, 1402 surgical patients were compared with 1489 contemporaneously matched controls who had declined an operation [82]. After 2 years, the mean body weight in the surgery group had dropped by 23.4% while in the control group it had increased by 0.1%. These changes were accompanied by a dramatic decrease in the incidence of T2DM in the surgical patients at 2 years (odds ratio, 0.14; 95% confidence interval [CI],

0.08–0.24) and at 10 years (odds ratio, 0.25; 95% CI, 0.17–0.38), confirming that bariatric surgery could prevent new-onset T2DM as well as reverse pre-existing disease. Schauer and colleagues [83] studied the preoperative predictors of T2DM resolution and confirmed that resolution was most likely to occur in patients with the mildest disease (oral medications; duration < 5 years) and the greatest weight loss. These findings have been confirmed by Torquati and colleagues [84] who also found peripheral fat distribution (small waist circumference) to be an independent predictor of T2DM resolution. Interestingly, the experience in adults is paralleled by the more limited studies available in adolescents. Complete resolution of T2DM has been reported in relatively small series by Sugerman and colleagues [85] and Fielding and Duncombe [86].

Other metabolic abnormalities are also responsive to bariatric procedures. Madan and colleagues [87] recently used NCEP-ATPIII criteria to identify 32 patients with the IRS and noted resolution in 31 patients following laparoscopic RYGB (96.8%). In two other studies, BPD was also shown to dramatically reverse IRS [88,89]. In addition, several other groups have evaluated patients with PCOS and documented significant improvements in the reproductive, metabolic, and cosmetic problems associated with this syndrome after bariatric procedures [90,91].

Similar benefits have been demonstrated using the LAGB, with T2DM remission rates reported to range from 64% to 71% within the first year [92,93]. Pontiroli and colleagues [94,95] studied a variety of clinical and metabolic factors in 143 morbidly obese patients treated by LAGB and compared them with a nonrandomized cohort of 120 equally obese control subjects. Following surgery, body fat distribution changed significantly, mostly due to the loss of visceral adiposity. This loss was accompanied by a rapid and sustained improvement in insulin resistance as measured by decreases in serum insulin levels and in the homeostasis model assessment (HOMA). During the same time, mean plasma glucose and hemoglobin A_{1c} (HbA$_{1c}$) levels normalized and dyslipidemias improved (Fig. 3). These postoperative changes were more evident in patients who had T2DM than in the impaired glucose tolerance group. Similarly, O'Brien and colleagues [75] reported a randomized, controlled study of 80 obese patients (BMI, 30–35) comparing LAGB with intensive medical therapy. The IRS was initially diagnosed in 15 patients in each group (38%). After 2 years, evidence for the IRS was still present in eight of the control patients (24%) but only one surgical patient (3%), and the quality of life was significantly better in the surgical group.

The cumulative experience with various operative techniques has been summarized in a recent meta-analysis of 22,094 morbidly obese patients by Buchwald and colleagues (Table 2) [96]. T2DM was diagnosed in 15.3% of the evaluable patients, and impaired glucose tolerance was diagnosed in 25.8%. Overall, T2DM resolved in 76.8% of all documented cases, with glycemic improvement observed in all types of bariatric surgery. Long-term survival was not addressed in this analysis and is not commonly

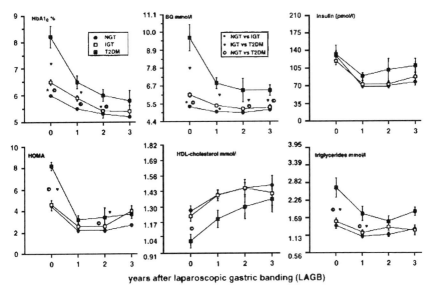

Fig. 3. Three-year behavior of HbA$_{1c}$, fasting blood glucose (BG) (mmol/L), fasting insulin (pmol/L), HOMA, HDL cholesterol (mmol/L), and triglycerides (mmol/L) in grade 3 obese patients with normal glucose tolerance (NGT), impaired glucose tolerance (IGT), and T2DM undergoing LAGB. Means ± SE. (*From* Pontiroli AE, Pizzocri P, Librenti MC, et al. Laparoscopic adjustable gastric banding for the treatment of morbid (grade 3) obesity and its metabolic complications: a three-year study. J Clin Endocrinol Metab 2002;87:3560; used with permission. Copyright © 2002, The Endocrine Society.)

reported. Nevertheless, an 89% reduction in the relative risk of death was noted in a 5-year study performed at McGill University in which 1035 RYGB patients were compared with 5746 age- and gender-matched, nonoperated, severely obese patients [97].

The mechanisms responsible for the postoperative reversal of insulin resistance and its related disorders remain controversial. Most available

Table 2
Results of different types of bariatric surgery expressed as mean values from meta-analysis of 22,094 patients

	Malabsorptive (DS, BDP)	Restrictive (band, VBG)	Combined (RYGB)
Weight loss (% excess)	72	50–69	68
Abnormality resolved			
T2DM	98%	48%–68%	84%
Hypertension	81%	38%–73%	75%
Dyslipidemia improved	100%	71%–81%	94%
Operative mortality	1.10%	0.1%	0.5%

Data from Buchwald H, Avidor Y, Braunwald E, et al. Bariatric surgery: a systematic review and meta-analysis. JAMA 2004;292:1724–37.

evidence suggests that the extreme reduction in calorie intake induced by restrictive and malabsorptive procedures is the major factor. Nonetheless, because most of the metabolic effects of surgery are observed long before substantial weight loss occurs, it has been suggested that changes in regulatory peptides must also contribute [98,99].

The most commonly proposed mechanism involves alterations in the enteroinsular axis, the signaling pathway between the gut and the pancreas that serves to enhance insulin secretion in response to a meal [100]. The most important of the insulin secretagogues (incretins) are glucose-dependent insulinotropic peptide (GIP) and glucose-like peptide 1 (GLP-1) (Table 3). Both peptides are secreted by specialized cells in the gut, GIP by K cells in the duodenum and GLP-1 by L cells in the terminal ileum and colon. Together, they are responsible for 40% to 50% of postprandial insulin secretion, and both exhibit trophic effects by stimulating beta-cell proliferation and inhibiting apoptosis [101]. Overactivity of the enteroinsular axis has been cited as one potential cause of hyperinsulinism and T2DM [102].

Peptide YY (PYY) is another insulin-sensitizing peptide that is secreted by L cells in the hindgut. It is primarily involved in appetite regulation by stimulation of specific receptors in the hypothalamus. Together with GLP-1, it functions as an "ileal brake" by slowing gastric emptying and prolonging intestinal transit. Grehlin is a novel gastric peptide with receptors in the hypothalamus. It is released principally in the preprandial state and serves as a stimulant of appetite and intestinal motility. It has also

Table 3
Gastrointestinal hormone changes after bariatric surgery and their effect on insulin secretion

Hormone	Cell type and their location in the gastrointestinal tract	Effect on insulin secretion	Changes induced by surgery			Other actions
			BPD	RYGB	LAGB	
Grehlin	X/A-like cells, stomach	↓	↑	↓↑	NC	Orexigenic, stimulates GH
GIP	K cells, foregut	↑	↓	↓	UNK	
GLP-1	L cells, hindgut	↑	↑	↑	UNK	Anorectic "ileal break"
PYY	L cells, hindgut	UNK	UNK	↑	UNK	Anorectic "ileal break"

Abbreviations: NC, no change; PYY, peptide YY; UNK, unknown.

been shown to inhibit insulin secretion, impair insulin sensitivity, block adiponectin release, and stimulate the secretion of growth hormone. Changes in enteroinsular signaling following RYGB or BPD are thought to occur for two reasons: (1) the secretory mucosa of the excluded stomach, duodenum, and jejunum remains unstimulated because of the absence of food; and (2) the secretory mucosa of the terminal ileum is excessively stimulated because of the increased presence of incompletely digested food.

The role of foregut exclusion has been studied extensively by Rubino and Marescaux [103] using nonobese diabetic Goto-Kakizaki rats. They bypassed the duodenum and jejunum with a Roux-en-Y gastrojejunal anastomosis and found significant improvement in fasting glycemia and glucose tolerance within 3 weeks. Because this model was not associated with weight loss, unidentified humoral or neural factors independent of weight loss were suspected. Numerous other investigators have studied specific peptides, but the available data are inconclusive. Because grehlin and GIP are primarily secreted by foregut mucosa, they are the peptides most likely to decrease after a bypass operation. In fact, grehlin levels have been reported to increase, decrease, or remain unaltered following RYGB, an inconsistency that precludes assigning a mechanistic role [104–106]. Alternatively, GIP values are generally decreased following RYGB, especially in the presence of T2DM, but the significance of this finding remains to be determined [107,108].

In the hind gut, the normal responses of PYY and GLP-1 to a meal are clearly exaggerated following RYGB [109,110]. It seems likely that these increases contribute to the enhanced satiety that is characteristic of RYGB, but their precise relationship to the observed change in insulin sensitivity remains speculative. In this regard, Strader and colleagues [111] studied rats in which a short segment of ileum was surgically transposed to jejunum to rapidly expose the ileal endocrine cells to undigested nutrients. They confirmed a marked increase in the synthesis and secretion of PYY and GLP-1 and found improved insulin sensitivity in a comparison with sham-operated controls. These investigators and others have concluded that gastrointestinal peptides have a crucial role in glucose homeostasis and recommend that further evaluation should continue.

Metabolic complications

The potential for metabolic/endocrine complications to develop as a result of weight loss surgery has only recently become evident. Endogenous hyperinsulinemic hypoglycemia with nesidioblastosis has been described in nine patients at variable time intervals after gastric bypass surgery. In one patient, multiple insulinomas were also found. All patients presented with symptoms of neuroglycopenia associated with hyperinsulinemia. Nesidioblastosis is a rare condition in which hypertrophy, hyperplasia of pancreatic islets, and neodifferentiation of islet of Langerhans cells from pancreatic exocrine duct epithelium are observed. It has been hypothesized that this phenomenon could be caused by hypersecretion of GLP-1, a known beta-cell trophic factor, as a result of the gastric bypass (Fig. 4) [111,112]. Asymptomatic hyperinsulinemic hypoglycemia can also occur after gastric banding and is reported in 3% to 4% of LAGB patients [112,113]. It has been hypothesized that the substantial weight loss after this procedure markedly reduces insulin resistance in the context of beta-cell hypertrophy and hyperfunction that are characteristic of obesity, and that this effect may cause asymptomatic hypoglycemia. No patient undergoing gastric banding has been diagnosed with nesidioblastosis, pointing to a different pathogenesis of the hypoglycemia after the two different bariatric surgeries.

Practical considerations

Bariatric surgery is always elective. Indeed, the best metabolic results are achieved when patients have been fully prepared and are adequately followed. In the preoperative period, most morbidly obese patients are already insulin resistant even though only a minority have T2DM. Accordingly, each patient should be assessed carefully for the presence of the IRS, and individual risk factors should be treated aggressively to minimize the risk of intraoperative and postoperative complications. In particular, if T2DM is present, good glycemic control should be achieved before the operation ($HbA_{1c} < 7.0$) because infectious complications are more likely to occur in patients who are poorly controlled [114].

In the immediate postoperative period, most T2DM patients can expect a rapid reduction in or even termination of their diabetic medications; however, there are no specific guidelines for exact dosage changes. Oral diabetic medications can usually be withheld immediately after operation, but the

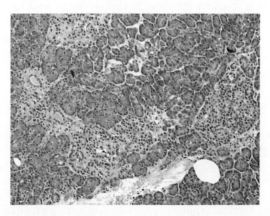

Fig. 4. Nesidioblastosis after gastric bypass surgery. There are several islets, some of which appear to be irregular and increased in size. Occasionally, groups of islets appear back-to-back close to small duct-forming structures resembling the ductuloinsular complexes. (Hematoxylin-eosin staining, final magnification ×200).

blood glucose levels should be carefully monitored and an insulin sliding scale initiated as necessary. Similarly, in patients who have more severe disease, such as those requiring insulin before surgery, a significant downward adjustment in medication dose is often possible before hospital discharge because considerable residual beta-cell function is usually present. In these patients, insulin needs should be managed initially with a sliding scale.

Following hospital discharge, caution is advisable in the use of antidiabetic medications because daily oral intake usually does not exceed 500 calories for the first 2 weeks. As intake gradually increases, efforts should be made to optimize protein intake and limit carbohydrate and fat calories. In addition, because insulin sensitivity is markedly influenced by physical activity, patients should be encouraged to begin an exercise regimen that is tailored to their individual abilities. A program of 30 minutes of moderate-intensity exercise 5 days each week will help to maximize weight loss, tone muscles, improve attitude, and avoid depression.

Summary

Insulin resistance is a nearly universal finding in morbid obesity. It may be compensated and latent or uncompensated with single or multiple clinical abnormalities, such as in the IRS, impaired glucose tolerance/T2DM, or PCOS. Although lifestyle interventions and medical measures alone may control most metabolic problems in the short term, the ultimate benefits of such an approach are usually limited by the complexity of available therapeutic regimens and the difficulty of maintaining full patient compliance. Many studies now document that bariatric surgery can effectively and safely control these complications in the short term and long term or even prevent their occurrence. Further investigations are needed to better understand the mechanisms involved and to define more clearly the appropriate indications and contraindications of the treatments proposed.

References

[1] Mokdad AH, Ford ES, Bowman BA, et al. Prevalence of obesity, diabetes, and obesity-related health risk factors, 2001. JAMA 2003;289:76–9.
[2] Zimmet P, Alberti KG, Shaw J. Global and societal implications of the diabetes epidemic. Nature 2001;414:782–7.
[3] American Diabetes Association. Economic costs of diabetes in the US in 2002. Diabetes Care 2003;26:917–32.
[4] Brown SA, Upchurch S, Anding R, et al. Promoting weight loss in type II diabetes. Diabetes Care 1996;19:613–24.
[5] Zimmet P, Shaw J, Alberti KG. Preventing type 2 diabetes and the dysmetabolic syndrome in the real world: a realistic view. Diabet Med 2003;20:693–702.
[6] Pories WJ, Swanson MS, MacDonald KG, et al. Who would have thought it? An operation proves to be the most effective therapy for adult-onset diabetes mellitus. Ann Surg 1995; 222:339–52.

[7] Saltiel AR, Kahn CR. Insulin signaling and the regulation of glucose and lipid metabolism. Nature 2001;414(6865):799–806.

[8] Caro JF, Ittoop O, Pories WJ, et al. Studies on the mechanism of insulin resistance in the liver from humans with noninsulin-dependent diabetes: insulin action and binding in isolated hepatocytes, insulin receptor structure, and kinase activity. J Clin Invest 1986; 78(1):249–58.

[9] Folli F, Saad MJA, Backer JM, et al. Regulation of phosphatidylinositol 3-kinase activity in liver and muscle of animal models of insulin resistant and insulin deficient diabetes mellitus. J Clin Invest 1993;92:1787–94.

[10] Rattarasarn C. Physiological and pathophysiological regulation of regional adipose tissue in the development of insulin resistance and type 2 diabetes. Acta Physiol 2006; 186:87–101.

[11] Abate N, Chandalia M, Di Paola R, et al. Mechanisms of disease: ectonucleotide pyrophosphatase phosphodiesterase 1 as a "gatekeeper" of insulin receptors. Nat Clin Pract Endocrinol Metab 2006;2(12):694–701.

[12] Almind K, Bjorbaek C, Vestergaard H, et al. Amino acid polymorphisms of insulin receptor substrate-1 in non–insulin-dependent diabetes mellitus. Lancet 1993;342(8875):828–32.

[13] Mayer EJ, Newman B, Austin MA, et al. Genetic and environmental influences on insulin levels and the insulin resistance syndrome: an analysis of women twins. Am J Epidemiol 1996;143:323–32.

[14] North KE, Williams K, Williams JT, et al. Evidence for genetic factors underlying the insulin resistance syndrome in American Indians. Obes Res 2003;11:1444–8.

[15] Moller N, Gormsen L, Fugisang J, et al. Effects of aging on insulin secretion and action. Horm Res 2003;60(Suppl 1):102–4.

[16] Stettler R, Ith M, Acheson KJ, et al. Interaction between dietary lipids and physical inactivity on insulin sensitivity and on intramyocellular lipids in healthy men. Diabetes Care 2005;28:1404–9.

[17] Pereira MA, Ludwig DS. Surveillance of insulin resistance in children. Clin Chem 2003;49: 540–1.

[18] Morino K, Petersen KF, Shulman GI. Molecular mechanisms of insulin resistance in humans and their potential links with mitochondrial dysfunction. Diabetes 2006;55(Suppl 2):S9–15.

[19] Kraegen EW, Cooney GJ, Ye JM, et al. The role of lipids in the pathogenesis of muscle insulin resistance and beta cell failure in type II diabetes and obesity. Exp Clin Endocrinol Diabetes 2001;109(Suppl 2):S189–201.

[20] Schrauwen-Hinderling VB, Hesselink MKC, Schrauwen P, et al. Intramyocellular lipid content in human skeletal muscle. Obesity 2006;14:357–67.

[21] Machann J, Haring H, Schick F, et al. Intramyocellular lipids and insulin resistance. Diabetes Obes Metab 2004;6:239–48.

[22] Kim JK, Gimeno RE, Higashimori T, et al. Inactivation of fatty acid transport protein 1 prevents fat-induced insulin resistance in skeletal muscle. J Clin Invest 2004;113:756–63.

[23] Theuma P, Fonseca VA. Inflammation and emerging risk factors in diabetes mellitus and atherosclerosis. Curr Diab Rep 2003;3:248–54.

[24] Wellen KE, Hotamisligil GS. Inflammation, stress and diabetes. J Clin Invest 2005;115: 1111–9.

[25] Ozcan U, Yilmaz E, Ozcan L, et al. Chemical chaperones reduce ER stress and restore glucose homeostasis in a mouse model of type 2 diabetes. Science 2006;313:1137–40.

[26] Furukawa S, Fujita T, Shimabukuro M, et al. Increased oxidative stress in obesity and its impact on metabolic syndrome. J Clin Invest 2004;114:1752–61.

[27] Furler SM, Gan SK, Poynten AM, et al. Relationship of adiponectin with insulin sensitivity in humans, independent of lipid availability. Obesity 2006;14:228–34.

[28] Gil-Campos M, Canete R, Gil A. Adiponectin, the missing link in insulin resistance and obesity. Clin Nutr 2004;23:963–74.

[29] Wiecek A, Kokot F, Chudek J, et al. The adipose tissue—a novel endocrine organ of interest to the nephrologist. Nephrol Dial Transplant 2002;17:191–5.

[30] Yamada T, Katagiri H, Ishigaki Y, et al. Signals from intra-abdominal fat modulate insulin and leptin sensitivity through different mechanisms: neuronal involvement in food-intake regulation. Cell Metab 2006;3:223–9.

[31] Szanto I, Kahn CR. Selective interaction between leptin and insulin signaling pathways in a hepatic cell line. Proc Nat Acad Sci 2000;97:2355–60.

[32] Carvalheira JB, Torsoni MA, Amaral ME, et al. Cross-talk between the insulin and leptin signaling systems in rat hypothalamus. Obes Res 2005;13:48–57.

[33] Muoio DM, Newgard CB. A is for adipokine. Nature 2005;436:337–8.

[34] Reaven GM. Role of insulin resistance in human disease (syndrome X): an expanded definition. Annu Rev Med 1993;44:121–31.

[35] Buse J, Cobin R, Coble Y, et al. ACE Position Statement. Endocr Pract 2003;9:240–52.

[36] Ahmed I, Goldstein BJ. Cardiovascular risk in the spectrum of type 2 diabetes mellitus [review]. Mt Sinai J Med 2006;73(5):759–68.

[37] Hulthe J, Bokemark LB, Wikstrand J, et al. The metabolic syndrome, LDL particle size, and atherosclerosis: the Atherosclerosis and Insulin Resistance (AIR) study. Arterioscler Thromb Vasc Biol 2000;20:2140–7.

[38] Depres JP, Lamache B, Mauriege P, et al. Hyperinsulinemia as an independent risk factor for ischemic heart disease. N Engl J Med 1996;334:952–7.

[39] Saely CH, Aczel S, Marte T, et al. The metabolic syndrome, insulin resistance, and cardiovascular risk in diabetic and nondiabetic patients. J Clin Endocrinol Metab 2005;90:5698–703.

[40] Reilly MP, Wolfe ML, Rhodes T, et al. Measures of insulin resistance add incremental value to the clinical diagnosis of metabolic syndrome in association with coronary atherosclerosis. Circulation 2004;110:803–9.

[41] DeFronzo RA, Ferrannini E. Insulin resistance: a multifaceted syndrome responsible for NIDDM, obesity, hypertension, dyslipidemia, and atherosclerotic cardiovascular disease. Diabetes Care 1991;14:173–94.

[42] Ilercil A, Devereux RB, Roman MJ, et al. Relationship of impaired glucose tolerance to left ventricular structure and function: the Strong Heart Study. Am Heart J 2001;141:992–8.

[43] Rutter MK, Parise H, Benjamin EJ, et al. Impact of glucose intolerance and insulin resistance on cardiac structure and function: sex-related differences in the Framingham Heart Study. Circulation 2003;107:448–54.

[44] Sharma S, Adrogue JV, Golfman L, et al. Intramyocardial lipid accumulation in the failing human heart resembles the lipotoxic rat heart. FASEB J 2004;18:1692–700.

[45] Reaven GM. The metabolic syndrome: is this diagnosis necessary? Am J Clin Nutr 2006;83:1237–47.

[46] Kahn R, Buse J, Ferrannini E, et al. The metabolic syndrome: time for a critical appraisal. Joint statement from the American Diabetes Association and the European Association for the Study of Diabetes. Diabetes Care 2005;28:2289–304.

[47] Grundy SM. Metabolic syndrome: connecting and reconciling cardiovascular and diabetes worlds. J Am Coll Cardiol 2006;47:1093–100.

[48] Grundy SM, Cleeman JI, Daniels SR, et al. Diagnosis and management of the metabolic syndrome: a statement for health professionals. An American Heart Association/National Heart Lung and Blood Institute Scientific statement. Circulation 2005;112:2735–52.

[49] Grundy S. Drug therapy of the metabolic syndrome: minimizing the emerging crisis in polypharmacy. Nature Rev 2006;5:295–309.

[50] Mattar S, Velcu L, Mordecai R, et al. Surgically induced weight loss significantly improves non-alcoholic fatty liver disease and the metabolic syndrome. Ann Surg 2005;242:610–20.

[51] DeFronzo RA. Pathogenesis of type 2 diabetes mellitus. Med Clin North Am 2004;88:787–835.

[52] Hu FB, Manson JE, Stampfer MJ, et al. Diet, lifestyle, and the risk of type 2 diabetes mellitus in women. N Engl J Med 2001;345:790–7.
[53] Willett WC, Dietz WH, Colditz GA. Guidelines for healthy weight. N Engl J Med 1999;141: 427–34.
[54] Kaufman FR. Diabesity. New York: Bantam Books; 2005.
[55] Fagot-Campagna A, Pettitt D, Engelgau MM, et al. Type 2 diabetes among North American children and adolescents: an epidemiological review and a public health perspective. J Pediatr 2000;236:664–72.
[56] Gu K, Cowie CC, Harris MI. Mortality in adults with and without diabetes in a national cohort of the US population, 1971–1993. Diabetes Care 1998;21:1138–45.
[57] Roglic G, Unwin N, Bennet PH, et al. The burden of mortality attributable to diabetes. Diabetes Care 2005;28:2130–5.
[58] Scheen AJ. Treatment of diabetes in patients with severe obesity. Biomed Pharmacother 2000;54:74–9.
[59] Campbell L, Rossner S. Management of obesity in patients with type 2 diabetes. Diabet Med 2001;18:345–54.
[60] Wing RR, Phelan S. Long-term weight loss maintenance. Am J Clin Nutr 2005;82(Suppl): 222S–5S.
[61] Sam S, Dunaif A. Polycystic ovary syndrome: syndrome XX. Trends Endocrinol Metab 2003;14:365–70.
[62] DeUgarte CM, Bartolucci AA, Azziz R. Prevalence of insulin resistance in the polycystic ovary syndrome using the homeostasis model assessment. Fertil Steril 2005;83:1454–60.
[63] Burghen GA, Givens JR, Kitabchi AD. Correlation of hyperandrogenism with hyperinsulinism in polycystic ovarian disease. J Clin Endocrinol Metab 1980;50:113–6.
[64] Legro RS, Gnatuk CL, Kunselman AR, et al. Changes in glucose tolerance over time in women with polycystic ovary syndrome: a controlled study. J Clin Endocrinol Metab 2005;90:3236–42.
[65] Cussons AJ, Stuckey BG, Watts GF. Cardiovascular disease in the polycystic ovary syndrome: new insights and perspectives. Atherosclerosis 2006;185:227–39.
[66] Hopkinson ZE, Sattar N, Fleming R, et al. Polycystic ovarian syndrome: the metabolic syndrome comes to gynaecology. BMJ 1998;317:329–32.
[67] Ehrmann DA. Polycystic ovary syndrome. N Engl J Med 2005;352:1223–36.
[68] Diamanti-Kandarakis E, Papavassiliou AG. Molecular mechanisms of insulin resistance in polycystic ovary syndrome. Trends Mol Med 2006;12:324–32.
[69] Kiddy DS, Hamilton-Fairley D, Bush A, et al. Improvement in endocrine and ovarian function during dietary treatment of obese women with polycystic ovary syndrome. Clin Endocrinol 1992;36:105–11.
[70] Lord JM, Flight IH, Norman RJ. Insulin-sensitizing drugs (metformin, troglitazone, rosiglitazone, pioglitazone, D-chiro-inositol) for polycystic ovary syndrome. Cochrane Database Syst Rev 2003;(2):CD003053.
[71] Hahn S, Benson S, Elsenbruch S, et al. Metformin treatment of polycystic ovary syndrome improves health-related quality-of-life, emotional distress and sexuality. Hum Reprod 2006;21:1925–34.
[72] Banaszewska B, Duleba AJ, Spaczynski RZ, et al. Lipids in polycystic ovary syndrome: role of hyperinsulinemia and effects of metformin. Am J Obstet Gynecol 2006;192:1266–72.
[73] National Institutes of Health Consensus Development Panel. Gastrointestinal surgery for severe obesity. Ann Intern Med 1991;115:956–61.
[74] Buchwald H. Consensus Conference Panel, bariatric surgery for morbid obesity: health implications for patients, health professionals, and third-party payers. J Am Coll Surg 2005;200:593–604.
[75] O'Brien PE, Dixon JB, Laurie C, et al. Treatment of mild to moderate obesity with laparoscopic adjustable gastric banding or an intensive medical program. Ann Intern Med 2006; 144:625–33.

[76] Greenway SE, Greenway FL, Klein S. Effects of obesity surgery on non-insulin-dependent diabetes mellitus. Arch Surg 2002;137:1109–17.
[77] Blackburn GL, Jones DB. Effective surgical treatment of diabetes for the obese patient. Curr Diab Rep 2006;6:85–7.
[78] Pinkney J, Kerrigan D. Current status of bariatric surgery in the treatment of type 2 diabetes. Obes Rev 2004;5:69–78.
[79] Jones DB, Provost DA, DeMaria EJ, et al. Optimal management of the morbidly obese patient: SAGES appropriateness conference statement. Surg Endosc 2004;18:1029–37.
[80] Fischer BL, Schauer P. Medical and surgical options in the treatment of severe obesity. Am J Surg 2002;184:9S–16S.
[81] MacDonald KG Jr, Long SD, Swanson MS, et al. The gastric bypass operation reduces the progression and mortality of non-insulin-dependent diabetes mellitus. J Gastrointest Surg 1997;1:213–20.
[82] Sjostrom L, Lindroos AK, Peltonen M, et al. Lifestyle, diabetes, and cardiovascular risk factors 10 years after bariatric surgery. N Engl J Med 2004;351:2683–93.
[83] Schauer PR, Burguera B, Ikramuddin S, et al. Effect of laparoscopic Roux-en-Y gastric bypass on type 2 diabetes mellitus. Ann Surg 2003;238:467–85.
[84] Torquati A, Lutfi R, Abumrad N, et al. Is Roux-en-Y gastric bypass surgery the most effective treatment for type 2 diabetes mellitus in morbidly obese patients? J Gastrointest Surg 2005;9:1112–8.
[85] Sugerman HJ, Sugerman EL, DeMaria EJ, et al. Bariatric surgery for severely obese adolescents. J Gastrointest Surg 2003;7:102–8.
[86] Fielding GA, Duncombe JE. Laparoscopic adjustable gastric banding in severely obese adolescents. Surg Obes Rel Dis 2005;1:399–407.
[87] Madan AK, Orth W, Ternovits CA, et al. Metabolic syndrome: yet another co-morbidity gastric bypass helps cure. Surg Obes Relat Dis 2006;2:48–51.
[88] Greco AV, Mingrone G, Giancaterini A, et al. Insulin resistance in morbid obesity: reversal with intramyocellular fat depletion. Diabetes 2002;51:144–51.
[89] Adami GF, Cordera R, Camerini G, et al. Long-term normalization of insulin sensitivity following biliopancreatic diversion for obesity. Int J Obes Relat Metab Disord 2004;28:671–3.
[90] Eid GM, Cottam DR, Velcu LM, et al. Effective treatment of polycystic ovarian syndrome with Roux-en-Y gastric bypass. Surg Obes Relat Dis 2005;1:77–80.
[91] Escobar-Morreale HF, Botella-Carretero JI, Alvarez-Blasco F, et al. The polycystic ovary syndrome associated with morbid obesity may resolve after weight loss induced by bariatric surgery. J Clin Endocrinol Metab 2005;90:6364–9.
[92] Dixon JB, O'Brien PE. Health outcomes of severely obese type 2 diabetic subjects 1 year after laparoscopic adjustable gastric banding. Diabetes Care 2002;25:358–63.
[93] Champault A, Duwat O, Polliand C, et al. Quality of life after laparoscopic gastric banding: prospective study with a follow-up of 2 years. Surg Laparosc Endosc Percutan Tech 2006;16:131–6.
[94] Pontiroli AE, Pizzocri P, Librenti MC, et al. Laparoscopic adjustable gastric banding for the treatment of morbid (grade 3) obesity and its metabolic complications: a three-year study. J Clin Endocrinol Metab 2002;87:3555–61.
[95] Pontiroli AE, Folli F, Paganelli M, et al. Laparoscopic gastric banding prevents type 2 diabetes and arterial hypertension, and induces their remission in morbid obesity: a 4-year controlled study. Diabetes Care 2005;28:2703–9.
[96] Buchwald H, Avidor Y, Braunwald E, et al. Bariatric surgery: a systematic review and meta-analysis. JAMA 2004;292:1724–37.
[97] Christou NV, Sampalis JS, Liberman M, et al. Surgery decreases long-term mortality, morbidity, and health care use in morbidly obese patients. Ann Surg 2004;240:416–24.
[98] Cummings DE, Overduin J, Foster-Schubert KE. Gastric bypass for obesity: mechanisms of weight loss and diabetes resolution. J Clin Endocrinol Metab 2004;89:2608–15.

[99] Ferchak CV, Meneghini LF. Obesity, bariatric surgery and type 2 diabetes—a systematic review. Diabetes Metab Res Rev 2004;20:438–45.

[100] Patriti A, Facchiano E, Sanna A, et al. The enteroinsular axis and the recovery from type 2 diabetes after bariatric surgery. Obes Surg 2004;14:840–8.

[101] Nauck MA, Meier JJ, Creutzfeldt W. Incretins and their analogues as new antidiabetic drugs [review]. Drug News Perspect 2003;16(7):413–22.

[102] Pories WJ. Diabetes: the evolution of a new paradigm. Ann Surg 2004;239:12–3.

[103] Rubino F, Marescaux J. Effect of duodenal-jejunal exclusion in a non-obese animal model of type 2 diabetes: a new perspective for an old disease. Ann Surg 2004;239:1–11.

[104] Cummings DE, Shannon MH. Grehlin and gastric bypass. Is there a hormonal contribution to surgical weight loss? J Clin Endocrinol Metab 2003;88:2999–3002.

[105] Korner J, Bessler M, Cirilo J, et al. Effects of Roux-en-Y gastric bypass surgery on fasting and postprandial concentrations of plasma ghrelin, peptide YY, and insulin. J Clin Endocrinol Metab 2005;90:359–65.

[106] Stratis C, Alexandrides T, Vagenas K, et al. Ghrelin and peptide YY levels after a variant of biliopancreatic diversion with Roux-en-Y gastric bypass versus after colectomy: a prospective comparative study. Obes Surg 2006;16:752–8.

[107] Sirinek KR, O'Dorisio TM, Hill D, et al. Hyperinsulinism, glucose-dependent insulinotropic polypeptide, and the enteroinsular axis in morbidly obese patients before and after gastric bypass. Surgery 1986;100:781–5.

[108] Guidone C, Manco M, Valera-Mora E, et al. Mechanisms of recovery from type 2 diabetes after malabsorptive bariatric surgery. Diabetes 2006;55:2025–31.

[109] le Roux CW, Aylwin SJ, Batterham RL, et al. Gut hormone profiles following bariatric surgery favor an anorectic state, facilitate weight loss, and improve metabolic parameters. Ann Surg 2006;243:108–14.

[110] Suzuki S, Ramos EJ, Goncalves DG, et al. Changes in GI hormones and the effect on gastric emptying and transit times after Roux-en-Y gastric bypass in rat model. Surgery 2005;138:283–90.

[111] Strader AD, Vahl TP, Jandacek RJ, et al. Weight loss through ileal transposition is accompanied by increased ileal hormone secretion and synthesis in rats. Am J Physiol Endocrinol Metab 2005;288:E447–53.

[112] Service GJ, Thompson GB, Service FJ, et al. Hyperinsulinemic hypoglycemia with nesidioblastosis after gastric-bypass surgery. N Engl J Med 2005;353:249–54.

[113] Scavini M, Pontiroli A, Folli F. Asymptomatic hyperinsulinemic hypoglycemia after laparoscopic adjustable gastric banding [letter to the editor]. N Engl J Med 2005;353:2822–3.

[114] Dronge AS, Perkal MF, Kancir S, et al. Long-term glycemic control and postoperative infectious complications. Arch Surg 2006;141:375–80.

ELSEVIER
SAUNDERS

THE MEDICAL
CLINICS
OF NORTH AMERICA

Med Clin N Am 91 (2007) 415–431

Impact of Obesity and Bariatric Surgery on Cardiovascular Disease

Michael A. Mathier, MD[a],
Ramesh C. Ramanathan, MD, FRCS[b],*

[a]UPMC Health System/Cardiovascular Institute, University of Pittsburgh School of
Medicine, 200 Lothrop Street, S 559 Scaife Hall, Pittsburgh, PA 15213, USA
[b]Magee Womens Hospital of UPMC, University of Pittsburgh School of Medicine,
Isaly's building, Suite 390, 3380 Boulevard of the Allies, Pittsburgh, PA 15213, USA

The prevalence of obesity is increasing rapidly and has become a major public health problem worldwide. More than half of the adult population in the United States is overweight or obese, and an estimated 5 to 10 million individuals are considered morbidly obese. With this increase in the prevalence of obesity has come an increase in the prevalence of heart disease. Studies indicate that body weight is an important independent predictor of the development of any heart disease and that its impact is felt disproportionately among women [1]. Obesity is associated particularly with an increased risk of heart failure: for each increment of 1 kg/m^2 in body mass index (BMI), there is a 5% increase in the risk of heart failure for men, and 7% for women [2].

Obesity leads to significant morbidity and mortality, and it is speculated that its increasing prevalence may begin to shorten overall life expectancy in the near future [3]. The morbidity and mortality rates rise proportionally to the degree of obesity, with a linear correlation demonstrated between BMI and mortality [4]. The risk of premature death in morbid obesity is doubled compared with nonobese individuals, and the risk of death from cardiovascular disease is increased fivefold [5].

Nonsurgical weight loss programs based on some combination of diet, exercise, and behavior modification commonly are ineffective in the long term [6]. Bariatric surgery offers an additional effective treatment option for long-term weight management for morbidly obese patients. In this article, we propose to review the current literature regarding the impact of obesity and bariatric surgery on cardiovascular disease.

* Corresponding author.
E-mail address: ramanathanrc@upmc.edu (R.C. Ramanathan).

Impact of obesity on cardiovascular risk factors and disease

It has become increasingly apparent that morbid obesity carries a heavy cardiovascular risk burden. Most cardiovascular risk factors and cardiovascular diseases occur with greater frequency and severity in patients who are morbidly obese. Given that cardiovascular disease represents by far the most common cause of serious morbidity and mortality in industrialized nations, the dramatic increase in obesity and morbid obesity seen over the last decade is clearly a profound public health concern [7].

The scope of cardiovascular risk factors and diseases impacted by obesity

Morbid obesity increases the frequency and severity of the metabolic syndrome, defined by the National Cholesterol Education Project Adult Treatment Panel III as the coexistence of any three of the following five features: central obesity, high serum triglyceride levels, low serum high-density lipoprotein (HDL)-cholesterol levels, hypertension, and elevated fasting blood glucose level. The metabolic syndrome is a potent risk factor for cardiovascular disease [8]. Related metabolic abnormalities commonly observed in obese patients include insulin resistance, hyperinsulinemia, and type 2 diabetes mellitus. Other risk factors for cardiovascular disease that are more prevalent in obese patients are obstructive sleep apnea and proinflammatory and prothrombotic states. Through these risk factors and independent of them, obesity increases the risk of the following cardiovascular diseases: systemic hypertension, coronary artery disease, heart failure, and cardiac dysrhythmias [9]. Each of these diseases is more difficult to treat when it occurs in the presence of morbid obesity, and the functional limitation imposed by each is more pronounced in morbidly obese patients.

Metabolic syndrome and its components

With the recent increase in rates of obesity and morbid obesity, a parallel increase in rates of metabolic syndrome has developed. The Third National Health and Nutrition Examination Survey (NHANES III) reported a nearly 24% prevalence of metabolic syndrome in US adults [10]. Disturbingly, there also appear to be rapid increases in its prevalence among children [11] and in countries in which it was until recently relatively uncommon [12]. Obesity, beyond being a cardinal feature of the metabolic syndrome, is also a critical trigger for it: a recent study suggested a prevalence of metabolic syndrome in obese patients that was nearly 10-fold higher than that in nonobese patients [13]. Obesity is so tightly linked with insulin resistance, hyperinsulinemia, and type 2 diabetes mellitus as to lead one group to discuss the global epidemic of "diabesity" [14]. In addition to the typical lipid abnormalities of elevated serum triglycerides and depressed serum HDL levels, obesity is also associated with elevated levels of oxidized low-density lipoprotein (LDL), an especially atherogenic lipoprotein [15]. Proinflammatory and prothrombotic states are common in patients with the metabolic syndrome (although uncommonly included in its definition) and also appear common in obese patients [16,17]. Recent evidence strongly suggests that the inflammatory aspects of obesity may be pivotal in the metabolic derangements that frequently ensue [18]. Inflammation and thrombosis now have well-established pathogenic links to many cardiovascular diseases.

Obstructive sleep apnea

Obese patients have a high prevalence of obstructive sleep apnea (OSA). Although it is estimated that 7% of all adults have significant OSA [19], the risk triples for each standard deviation increase in BMI [20]. The prevalence of OSA in patients undergoing evaluation for bariatric surgery may approach 80% [21]. Obstructive sleep apnea has numerous adverse sequelae, including associations with several cardiovascular diseases, including systemic and pulmonary hypertension, coronary artery disease, heart failure, stroke, and atrial fibrillation [22].

Hypertension

Systemic hypertension, like obesity and metabolic syndrome, has reached epidemic proportions in the United States. There is a clear link between obesity and hypertension, with data from NHANES III indicating an approximately threefold increase in the prevalence of hypertension in obese versus lean patients [23]. Although OSA appears to confer much of this increased risk [22], other mechanisms, including direct hemodynamic alterations, inflammation, and neurohormonal activation likely also play a role.

Coronary artery disease

Given the tight associations between obesity, the metabolic syndrome, and hypertension, and the potent risk conferred by the metabolic syndrome and hypertension for the development of atherosclerosis, it is unsurprising that obesity is associated with an increased prevalence of coronary artery disease. Pathological studies have shown an association between obesity early in life and the formation of atherosclerotic lesions [24]. A number of studies have documented a clear association between obesity and clinically manifest coronary artery disease [16]. Furthermore, the diagnostic evaluation of these patients and their subsequent revascularization by either percutaneous or surgical means can be a challenge. Most recent data have suggested, however, that current diagnostic tools and revascularization techniques are safe and effective in this population [25–28].

Heart failure

In the general population, longstanding obesity is a risk factor for heart failure even in the absence of traditional risk factors for coronary artery disease [29]. Over time, morbid obesity results in structural myocardial changes, including increased left ventricular (LV) dimensions and mass, and impaired LV relaxation and systolic function [30]. The mechanisms underlying these changes are not well understood but likely include altered loading conditions related to associated comorbidities such as hypertension and OSA, insulin resistance, and abnormal neurohormonal and cytokine profiles. Surprisingly, despite being a risk factor for the development of heart failure, data suggest that obesity is protective in patients with established heart failure [31], a phenomenon termed *the obesity paradox*. This observation has not thus far been extended to morbidly obese patients. Both morbid obesity and heart failure markedly reduce functional capacity [32], and patients with the combination of the two conditions have severe functional limitation and poor survival. In addition, the presence of advanced heart failure makes weight loss by conventional means nearly impossible for these patients. Finally, the presence of morbid obesity generally disqualifies patients from consideration for cardiac transplantation.

Cardiac dysrhythmias

Obesity increases the risk of cardiac dysrhythmias, including atrial fibrillation [33–35], ventricular ectopy, and sudden cardiac death [36,37]. There are numerous potential explanations for this association. Obesity is, again, associated with hypertension, OSA, coronary artery disease and its risk factors, and changes in cardiac structure and function, all of which are independent risk factors for cardiac dysrhythmias. More mechanistically, obesity has been shown to be associated with abnormalities in cardiac repolarization, as evidenced by prolongation of the QT interval and by an increase in late potentials [38,39]. In addition, pathological abnormalities of the cardiac conduction system have been observed in obese patients after sudden cardiac death [40].

Stroke

Obesity has been shown recently to increase the risk of both ischemic and hemorrhagic stroke, independent of associated conditions known to increase stroke risk (metabolic syndrome, hypertension, OSA) [41]. In this study, obese male patients faced twice the risk of stroke as did their lean counterparts, and each one-unit increase in BMI over 25 kg/m^2 increased the risk of stroke by approximately 5%. The mechanisms for this independent association are not completely known but likely involve inflammatory and thrombotic pathways.

Impact of obesity on cardiac structure and function

Chronic obesity is associated with changes in cardiac structure and function, which appear to be dependent on both the severity and the duration of obesity [30]. Left ventricular hypertrophy and increased cardiac mass generally are observed in obese patients, and measures of diastolic left ventricular function often are abnormal, even in the absence of overt heart failure [42]. Left [30] and right [43] ventricular dilatation and impaired systolic function may also occur in obese patients. Fatty infiltration of the heart (adipositas cordis) has been reported in obese patients and may contribute to the abnormalities of cardiac structure and function observed [5]. Hemodynamic alterations are known to exist in obese patients, primarily increased cardiac output and filling pressures. The mechanisms of altered cardiac structure and function in obesity may include altered hemodynamic load, metabolic abnormalities, inflammation, coronary artery disease, and, perhaps, direct myocardial effects of adipocyte-related hormones.

Effects of bariatric surgery on cardiovascular risk factors

Numerous studies have documented the beneficial impact of weight loss on most cardiovascular risk factors. Given the high rate of successful weight reduction with bariatric surgery, it is unsurprising that the literature is replete with studies documenting its favorable impact on these risk factors

Metabolic syndrome and its components

Bariatric surgery results in complete resolution or significant improvement in type 2 diabetes in the overwhelming majority of patients; this reached 86% in one study of patients followed up for 7 years after gastric bypass [44]. In a meta-analysis of 136 studies, nearly 77% of patients had resolution of type 2 diabetes after bariatric surgery [45]. The rate of resolution seemed to vary depending on the type of surgery, with combined restrictive or malabsorptive procedures having a higher rate of resolution compared with purely restrictive procedures. This effect appears to be durable, with one study finding an 83% resolution rate at 14 years after gastric bypass [46]. This durability, however, is dependant on maintenance of weight loss for the long term. In the Swedish obesity study, the resolution rate of type 2 diabetes decreased from 72% at 2 years to 36% at 10 years, with the recurrence being accompanied by a significant increase in body weight [47].

Significant improvements in lipid profiles after bariatric surgery have been shown in several studies, including reductions in total cholesterol, LDL cholesterol, and triglycerides and increases in HDL cholesterol. Improvements occur in more than 70% of patients, with the maximum improvement occurring after malabsorptive surgical procedures [45]. In a more integrated analysis, Lee and colleagues [48] reported a nearly 96%

resolution of metabolic syndrome associated with significant weight loss 1 year after bariatric surgery.

Obstructive sleep apnea

Surgical weight loss results in resolution of OSA and obesity hypoventilation syndrome in approximately 85% of patients [45]. Significant improvement in cardiac dysrhythmias associated with OSA has also been shown after gastric bypass surgery [49].

Hypertension

Intentional weight loss, both dietary and surgical, results in reductions in blood pressure, with a 1% decrease in body weight being associated with an approximate 1 mm Hg decrease in systolic blood pressure and an approximate 2 mm Hg decrease in diastolic blood pressure [50]. In a series of 1025 patients undergoing gastric bypass surgery, a 69% resolution of hypertension at 1 year and 66% resolution at 7 years were found [44]. The rate of complete resolution or significant improvement of hypertension was 79% in a meta-analysis of 136 studies relating to obesity surgery [45]. Interestingly, in the Swedish obesity study the 2- and 10-year resolution rates for hypertension after obesity surgery (34% and 19%, respectively) were much lower, although still better than the resolution rates in control subjects (21% and 11%, respectively) [47]. This may be a reflection of the poor weight loss results achieved in this study in which the majority of the patients underwent a restrictive surgical procedure (vertical banded gastroplasty), which is known to have a significant failure rate and weight recidivism.

Bariatric surgery in patients with cardiovascular disease

Bariatric surgery can be performed safely in patients with preexisting cardiovascular disease. In a study comparing outcomes of bariatric surgery in 52 patients with coronary artery disease (CAD) and 507 patients without CAD, a modest increase in the incidence of nonfatal cardiovascular events was observed in CAD patients (5.8% versus 1.4%) with no increase in mortality rate [51]. After a mean follow-up of 2.5 years, 63% of patients achieved more than 50% excess weight loss, with an accompanying major improvement in several risk factors linked to cardiovascular disease. In a retrospective analysis of 77 morbidly obese patients with preexisting cardiac disease (45 with coronary artery disease, 32 with heart failure), Roux-en-Y gastric bypass was performed with acceptable morbidity and excellent results [52]. We recently reported our outcomes from bariatric surgery in 14 morbidly obese patients with severe heart failure and left ventricular ejection fraction of ≤35% [53]. There was no mortality and acceptable morbidity with a median hospital length of stay of 3 days.

Although bariatric surgery can be performed safely in patients with pre-existing cardiovascular disease, many of these patients are at significant risk for peri- and post-operative complications. They should be managed by a multidisciplinary team, with a thorough preoperative evaluation, optimization of cardiovascular status, and careful perioperative monitoring.

Effect of bariatric surgery on cardiovascular disease

Several randomized, controlled trials have found that multiple risk factor reduction programs coupled with weight reduction result in slower progression or regression of anatomic CAD and decreased anginal symptoms [54,55]. In the Framingham cohort, a 10% reduction in body weight resulted in a 20% decrease in the risk of cardiovascular disease [56]. Furthermore, it is well established that improvements in risk factor profiles in patients with established CAD result in decreased rates of progression of atherosclerosis and reduced cardiac hospitalizations [57]. It should follow that bariatric surgery, which results in significant improvements in cardiovascular risk factor profiles, should have a beneficial effect on cardiovascular morbidity and mortality. Support for this idea is lent by the Program On the Surgical Control of the Hyperlipidemias (POSCH) trial, in which patients who had a partial ileal bypass showed a 23% decrease in total cholesterol levels and a 38% decrease in LDL cholesterol levels, resulting in a 60% decrease in the need for coronary intervention and a 20% reduction in the risk of mortality at a mean follow-up of 18 years [58].

Coronary artery disease

Bariatric surgery appears to slow the progression of atherosclerotic disease. In a study of carotid artery atherosclerosis in 20 patients treated with gastroplasty and 19 obese patients treated with dietary recommendations, the rate of progression was three-fold higher in controls compared with patients in the surgical group [59]. In a large observational cohort study, the incidence of coronary events (angina, myocardial infarction, and pulmonary edema) over a 5-year follow-up period was significantly reduced in patients undergoing bariatric surgery compared with controls. In addition, the number of percutaneous and surgical revascularization procedures was significantly lower in the surgical group [60].

Heart failure

Although a number of studies have examined the impact of bariatric surgery on the abnormalities of cardiac structure and function that accompany morbid obesity, few have documented its impact on the clinical syndrome of heart failure. We have recently reported beneficial effects of bariatric surgery in a cohort of morbidly obese patients with severe systolic LV failure.

Improvements in NYHA functional class and LV ejection fraction were noted at 6 and 12 months of follow-up compared with age, sex, ejection fraction and BMI matched controls [61].

Cardiac dysrhythmias and stroke

No reports exist as to the impact of bariatric surgery on the risk of cardiac dysrhythmia or stroke. A small, uncontrolled study of patients undergoing vertical banded gastroplasty noted a significant reduction in the corrected QT interval on follow-up 8 to 10 months after surgery, leading the investigators to speculate that this might decrease the risk of ventricular dysrhythmias [62].

Overall mortality

Several recent studies have indicated a survival advantage for patients undergoing bariatric surgery compared with control groups. In the Swedish obesity study, the adjusted overall mortality rate was reduced by 32% in the surgical group. The decrease in mortality was comprised of reductions in both cardiovascular and cancer deaths [63]. A more recent analysis compared a surgical cohort of 1468 patients undergoing laparoscopic adjustable gastric banding to a cohort of more than 2000 obese controls and found a 73% reduction in the mortality rate in the surgical group [64]. In the largest comparative study to date, 8172 patients who had undergone gastric bypass surgery were followed up for up to 18 years and found to have a 40% reduction in mortality rate compared with controls matched for age, sex, and BMI. This survival advantage was again associated with reductions in cardiovascular and cancer deaths [65].

Effects of bariatric surgery on cardiac structure and function

A number of studies have examined the effect of weight loss on cardiac structure and function, only a few of which have evaluated the effects of diet-induced weight loss. A randomized, controlled trial of weight reduction through diet and exercise in obese patients resulted in significant reductions in left ventricular hypertrophy and mass [66]. In an uncontrolled study of diet and exercise-induced weight loss in obese women, BMI, blood pressure, and cardiac output all decreased significantly, whereas markers of compliance improved [67]. Short and longer-term diet and exercise weight loss programs also have been shown to decrease heart rate and enhance parasympathetic cardiac tone [68,69].

Several studies have assessed the effects of surgically induced weight loss on cardiac structure and function, a number of which have been previously reviewed [5]. The results from five of these studies are summarized in Table 1 [70–75]. As can be seen, substantial weight loss through surgical intervention

Table 1
Effects of surgically induced weight loss on cardiac structure and function

Study	N	Preop weight (kg)	Preop BMI	Surgical procedure	Follow-up (mo)	Postop weight (kg)	Postop BMI (kg/m²)	Cardiac assessment: observations
Alpert, 1985 [70]	34	135 ± 8	—	Gastric restriction	4.3 ± 0.3	79 ± 6	—	Echo: LVFS% increase, LVIDD decrease (in subset (n = 13) with preop LV dysfunction)
Sugerman, 1988 [71]	18	[% IBW 225 ± 46]	—	Various	3–9	[% IBW 167 ± 57]	—	RHC: PAP decrease, PAOP decrease
Karason, 1997 & 1998 [72,73]	41	117 ± 15	39 ± 4	"Weight-reducing gastric surgery"	12	84 ± 14	29 ± 3	Echo: CO decrease, E/A increase, LVEF increase, LVM decrease, relative WT decrease
Kanoupakis, 2001 [74]	16	139 ± 24	49 ± 8	Vertical banded gastroplasty	6	94 ± 24	34 ± 7	ETT: peak VO$_2$ increase Echo: LV wall thickness decrease, IVRT decrease, E/A increase
Willens, 2005 [75]	17	160 ± 43	54 ± 11	Roux-en-Y gastric bypass	7.6 ± 3.6	121 ± 43	40 ± 11	Echo: LVM decrease, mitral and tricuspid annular early diastolic velocity increase

Abbreviations: CO, cardiac output; E/A, ratio of transmitral early to atrial peak flow velocity; Echo, echocardiogram; IBW, ideal body weight; IVRT, isovolumic relaxation time; LVEF, left ventricular ejection fraction; LVFS, left ventricular fractional shortening; LVIDD, left ventricular internal dimension in diastole; LVM, left ventricular mass; PAP, pulmonary artery occlusion pressure; PAP, pulmonary artery pressure; Relative WT, ratio of mean left ventricular wall thickness to left ventricular chamber radius; RHC, right heart catheterization; VO$_2$, oxygen consumption.

consistently results in improved left ventricular hypertrophy and frequently in improved measures of systolic and diastolic performance. One weakness of most studies published to date is the absence of an appropriate control group. Of note, however, Karason and colleagues [72,73] included as control groups in their study patients who were obese and received only dietary counseling and patients who were lean. In neither control group did body weight or cardiac parameters change during the study period. A more integrated view of the effects of bariatric surgery may come from measures of exercise performance. In a study of 31 morbidly obese patients undergoing bariatric surgery, substantial weight reduction resulted in a decrease in oxygen use per unit of work and an increase in total exercise time [76]. No changes in cardiac function were observed after surgery, however, emphasizing the importance of noncardiac factors in determining exercise performance, especially after the dramatic physiologic changes induced by profound weight loss.

Putative mechanisms for the cardiovascular effects of bariatric surgery

A number of putative mechanisms have been put forward to explain the beneficial effects of weight loss on cardiac structure and function. These include improvements in loading conditions, neurohormonal and metabolic profiles, and circulating levels of proinflammatory cytokines and markers of the systemic inflammatory state. Similar mechanistic explanations have been advanced to explain the benefits of the procedure on cardiovascular risk factors and manifest cardiovascular disease. One potential added mechanism is alterations in the expression of adipokines such as leptin and adiponectin, which have recently been shown to have direct effect on cardiac and vascular structure and function.

Altered loading conditions

Loading conditions are improved in obese patients after weight loss in a number of ways: via decreased circulating blood volume, cardiac output, intracardiac filling pressures, and systemic and pulmonary arterial pressure. The improvement in OSA usually seen after weight loss likely contributes to several of these changes. Interestingly, decreases in LV mass after weight loss appear to be largely independent of decreases in systemic arterial pressure [77], raising the likelihood that other mechanisms are at play. Neurohormonal activation, most notably of the sympathetic nervous system, is improved after weight loss [78] and might be expected to contribute to improvements in LV structure and function. Inflammatory and prothrombotic markers are similarly improved [79]. There is now ample evidence that inflammation contributes to many types of cardiovascular pathophysiology [80]. Again, the improvement in OSA that follows weight reduction likely contributes to these improvements in neurohormonal and inflammatory profiles [81].

Altered adipokine profile

Weight loss in obese patients is associated with partial normalization in circulating levels of adipokines, including leptin and adiponectin [82]. Emerging data suggest that these changes may play a role in the improvements seen in cardiovascular risk factors, cardiac structure and function, and clinical cardiovascular disease. Precise mechanisms, however, remain uncertain.

Leptin is a cytokine produced primarily by adipocytes; it acts via hypothalamic pathways to suppress appetite and increase metabolic rate [83]. Serum leptin levels are increased in obesity, although experimental work, coupled with the observation that appetite and metabolic parameters do not normalize in many obese patients despite high circulating leptin levels, raises the speculation that human obesity is a leptin-resistant state [84].

Leptin has been found to have direct cardiac and vascular effects, and leptin receptors are found in both cardiac [85] and vascular [86] tissue. Interestingly, leptin levels are elevated in nonobese patients after myocardial infarction [87] and in the presence of heart failure [88]. Conflicting data exist as to the effect of leptin on cardiac hypertrophy, suggesting a complex relationship between leptin, its determinants, and cardiac mass [89,90]. Leptin levels have been found to decrease after bariatric surgery and to correlate with reductions in left ventricular hypertrophy [91]. High circulating leptin levels have been shown to be an independent risk factor for coronary artery disease [92] and for restenosis after coronary stenting [93]. Paradoxically, leptin signaling appears to be protective in experimental models of ischemia-reperfusion [94,95], suggesting differential effects of leptin according to experimental setting, site of action, or the specific disease state.

Adiponectin is also a cytokine produced by adipocytes but, in contrast to leptin, its plasma levels are significantly reduced in obesity. Adiponectin appears to exert insulin sensitizing and anti-inflammatory effects, and to have a protective effect against atherogenesis [96]. Clinical studies have found a relationship between low serum levels of adiponectin and increased risk of new-onset insulin resistance [97] and type 2 diabetes [98]. Although some studies have found an inverse relationship between serum adiponectin concentration and subsequent risk of myocardial infarction [99], others have found no relationship between the two [100]. The presence of adiponectin has been found to correlate positively with mortality in patients with chronic heart failure [101], perhaps reflecting the wasting condition known to be associated with poor prognosis in these patients. Interestingly, treatment of patients with type 2 diabetes with an angiotensin-converting enzyme inhibitor increased vascular adiponectin gene expression and improved endothelial function [102]. Bariatric surgery has also been shown to increase adiponectin levels [103], although the relationship between the increase and the beneficial cardiovascular effects of weight loss induced by the surgery has not been definitively established.

Summary

Morbid obesity is a growing public health concern with multiple associated cardiovascular comorbidities. Bariatric surgery has emerged as a safe and effective treatment for morbidly obese patients at risk for, or already suffering from, cardiovascular disease. Weight loss induced by the surgery has been shown to improve cardiovascular risk factors, cardiac structure and function, and the clinical course of established cardiovascular disease. The role of adipocyte-derived cytokines in mediating cardiovascular pathophysiology in obesity—and its modulation after weight loss—is under active investigation.

References

[1] Hubert HB, Feinleib M, McNamara PM, et al. Obesity as an independent risk factor for cardiovascular disease: a 26 year follow-up of participants in the Framingham heart study. Circulation 1983;67(5):968–77.
[2] Kenchaiah S, Evans JC, Levy D, et al. Obesity and the risk of heart failure. N Engl J Med 2002;347(5):305–13.
[3] Olshansky SJ, Passaro DJ, Hershow RC, et al. A potential decline in life expectancy in the United States in the 21st century. N Engl J Med 2005;352:1138–45.
[4] Calle EE, Thun MJ, Petrelli JM, et al. Body-mass index and mortality in a prospective cohort of U.S. adults. N Engl J Med 1999;341(15):1097–105.
[5] Poirier P, Martin J, Marceau P, et al. Impact of bariatric surgery on cardiac structure, function and clinical manifestations in morbid obesity. Expert Rev Cardiovasc Ther 2004;2(2): 193–201.
[6] Klein S, Burke LE, Bray GA, et al, American Heart Association Council on Nutrition, Physical Activity, and Metabolism. Clinical implications of obesity with specific focus on cardiovascular disease: a statement for professionals from the American Heart Association Council on Nutrition, Physical Activity, and Metabolism: endorsed by the American College of Cardiology Foundation. Circulation 2004;110:2952–67.
[7] Poirier P, Giles TD, Bray GA, et al. Obesity and cardiovascular disease: pathophysiology, evaluation, and effect of weight loss: an update of the 1997 American Heart Association Scientific Statement on Obesity and Heart Disease from the Obesity Committee of the Council on Nutrition, Physical Activity, and Metabolism. Circulation 2006;113:898–918.
[8] Lakka HM, Laaksonen DE, Lakka TA, et al. The metabolic syndrome and total and cardiovascular disease mortality in middle-aged men. JAMA 2002;288:2709–16.
[9] Murphy NF, MacIntyre K, Stewart S, et al. Long-term cardiovascular consequences of obesity: 20-year follow-up of more than 15 000 middle-aged men and women (the Renfrew-Paisley study). Eur Heart J 2006;27:96–106.
[10] Ford ES, Giles WH, Dietz WH. Prevalence of the metabolic syndrome among US adults: findings from the third National Health and Nutrition Examination Survey. JAMA 2002; 287:356–9.
[11] Braunschweig CL, Gomez S, Liang H, et al. Obesity and risk factors for the metabolic syndrome among low-income, urban, African American schoolchildren: the rule rather than the exception? Am J Clin Nutr 2005;81:970–5.

[12] Gu D, Reynolds K, Wu X, et al. Prevalence of the metabolic syndrome and overweight among adults in China. Lancet 2005;365:1398–405.
[13] Meigs JB, Wilson PW, Fox CS, et al. Body mass index, metabolic syndrome, and risk of type 2 diabetes or cardiovascular disease. J Clin Endocrinol Metab 2006;91:2906–12.
[14] Zimmet P, Alberti KG, Shaw J. Global and societal implications of the diabetes epidemic. Nature 2001;414:782–7.
[15] Weinbrenner T, Schroder H, Escurriol V, et al. Circulating oxidized LDL is associated with increased waist circumference independent of body mass index in men and women. Am J Clin Nutr 2006;83:30–5.
[16] Grundy SM. Obesity, metabolic syndrome, and cardiovascular disease. J Clin Endocrinol Metab 2004;89:2595–600.
[17] Kahn SE, Zinman B, Haffner SM, et al, ADOPT Study Group. Obesity is a major determinant of the association of C-reactive protein levels and the metabolic syndrome in type 2 diabetes. Diabetes 2006;55:2357–64.
[18] Shoelson SE, Lee J, Goldfine AB. Inflammation and insulin resistance. J Clin Invest 2006; 116:1793–801.
[19] Young T, Peppard PE, Gottlieb DJ. Epidemiology of obstructive sleep apnea: a population health perspective. Am J Respir Crit Care Med 2002;165:1217–39.
[20] Young T, Palta M, Dempsey J, et al. The occurrence of sleep-disordered breathing among middle-aged adults. N Engl J Med 1993;328:1230–5.
[21] O'Keeffe T, Patterson EJ. Evidence supporting routine polysomnography before bariatric surgery. Obes Surg 2004;14:23–6.
[22] Quan SF, Gersh BJ. Cardiovascular consequences of sleep-disordered breathing: past, present and future: report of a workshop from the National Center on Sleep Disorders Research and the National Heart, Lung, and Blood Institute. Circulation 2004;109:951–7.
[23] Brown CD, Higgins M, Donato KA, et al. Body mass index and the prevalence of hypertension and dyslipidemia. Obes Res 2000;8:605–19.
[24] McGill HC Jr, McMahan CA, Herderick EE, et al. Obesity and atherosclerosis in youth. Circulation 2002;105:2712–8.
[25] Duvall WL, Croft LB, Corriel JS, et al. SPECT myocardial perfusion imaging in morbidly obese patients: image quality, hemodynamic response to pharmacologic stress, and diagnostic and prognostic value. J Nucl Cardiol 2006;13:202–9.
[26] McNulty PH, Ettinger SM, Field JM, et al. Cardiac catheterization in morbidly obese patients. Catheter Cardiovasc Interv 2002;56:174–7.
[27] Jin R, Grunkemeier GL, Furnary AP, et al. Is obesity a risk factor for mortality in coronary artery bypass surgery? Circulation 2005;111:3359–65.
[28] Nikolsky E, Kosinski E, Mishkel GJ, et al. Impact of obesity on revascularization and restenosis rates after bare-metal and drug-eluting stent implantation (from the TAXUS-IV trial). Am J Cardiol 2005;95:709–15.
[29] Wison PW, D'Agostino RB, Sullivan L, et al. Overweight and obesity as determinants of cardiovascular risk: the Framingham experience. Arch Intern Med 2002;162:1867–72.
[30] Alpert MA, Lambert CR, Panayiotou H, et al. Relation of duration of morbid obesity to left ventricular mass, systolic function, diastolic filling, and effect of weight loss. Am J Cardiol 1995;76:1194–7.
[31] Lavie CJ, Osman AF, Milani RV, et al. Body composition and prognosis in chronic systolic heart failure: the obesity paradox. Am J Cardiol 2003;99:891–4.
[32] Gallagher MJ, Franklin BA, Ehrman JK, et al. Comparative impact of morbid obesity vs heart failure on cardiorespiratory fitness. Chest 2005;127:2197–203.
[33] Dublin S, French B, Glazer NL, et al. Risk of new-onset atrial fibrillation in relation to body mass index. Arch Intern Med 2006;166:2322–8.
[34] Wang TJ, Parise H, Levy D, et al. Obesity and the risk of new-onset atrial fibrillation. JAMA 2004;292:2471–7.

[35] Zacharias A, Schwann TA, Riordan CJ, et al. Obesity and risk of new-onset atrial fibrillation after cardiac surgery. Circulation 2005;112:3247–55.

[36] Messerli FH, Nunez BD, Ventura HO, et al. Overweight and sudden death: increased ventricular ectopy in cardiomyopathy of obesity. Arch Intern Med 1987;147:1725–8.

[37] Duflou J, Virmani R, Rabin I, et al. Sudden death as a result of heart disease in morbid obesity. Am Heart J 1995;130:306–13.

[38] el-Gamal A, Gallagher D, Nawras A, et al. Effects of obesity on QT, RR, and QTc intervals. Am J Cardiol 1995;75:956–9.

[39] Lalani AP, Kanna B, John J, et al. Abnormal signal-averaged electrocardiogram (SAECG) in obesity. Obes Res 2000;8:20–8.

[40] Bharati S, Lev M. Cardiac conduction system involvement in sudden death of obese young people. Am Heart J 1995;129:273–81.

[41] Kurth T, Gaziano JM, Berger K, et al. Body mass index and the risk of stroke in men. Arch Intern Med 2002;162:2557–62.

[42] Zarich SW, Kowalchuk GJ, McGuire MP, et al. Left ventricular filling abnormalities in asymptomatic morbid obesity. Am J Cardiol 1991;68:377–81.

[43] Alpert MA, Singh A, Terry BE, et al. Effect of exercise and cavity size on right ventricular function in morbid obesity. Am J Cardiol 1989;64:1361–5.

[44] Sugerman HJ, Wolfe LG, Sica DA, et al. Diabetes and hypertension in severe obesity and effects of gastric bypass-induced weight loss. Ann Surg 2003;237(6):751–6.

[45] Buchwald H, Avidor Y, Braunwald E, et al. Bariatric surgery: a systematic review and meta-analysis. JAMA 2004;292(14):1724–37.

[46] Pories WJ, Swanson MS, MacDonald KG, et al. Who would have thought it? An operation proves to be the most effective therapy for adult-onset diabetes mellitus. Ann Surg 1995;222(3):339–50.

[47] Sjostrom L, Lindroos AK, Peltonen M, et al. Lifestyle, diabetes, and cardiovascular risk factors 10 years after bariatric surgery. N Engl J Med 2004;351(26):2683–93.

[48] Lee WJ, Huang MT, Wang W, et al. Effects of obesity surgery on the metabolic syndrome. Arch Surg 2004;139(10):1088–92.

[49] Peiser J, Ovnat A, Uwyyed K, et al. Cardiac arrhythmias during sleep in morbidly obese sleep-apneic patients before and after gastric bypass surgery. Clin Cardiol 1985;8(10):519–21.

[50] Bouldin MJ, Ross LA, Sumrall CD, et al. The effect of obesity surgery on obesity comorbidity. Am J Med Sci 2006;331(4):183–93.

[51] Lopez-Jimenez F, Bhatia S, Collazo-Clavell ML, et al. Safety and efficacy of bariatric surgery in patients with coronary artery disease. Mayo Clin Proc 2005;80(9):1157–62.

[52] Alsabrook GD, Goodman HR, Alexander JW. Gastric bypass for morbidly obese patients with established cardiac disease. Obes Surg 2006;16(10):1272–7.

[53] McCloskey CA, Ramani G, Mathier M, et al. Bariatric surgery in patients with cardiomyopathy. Surg Obes Relat Dis 2006;2(3):295.

[54] Niebauer J, Hambrecht R, Velich T, et al. Attenuated progression of coronary artery disease after 6 years of multifactorial risk intervention: role of physical exercise. Circulation 1997;96(8):2534–41.

[55] Ornish D, Brown SE, Scherwitz LW, et al. Can lifestyle changes reverse coronary heart disease? The lifestyle heart trial. Lancet 1990;336(8708):129–33.

[56] Gordon T, Kannel WB. Obesity and cardiovascular diseases: the Framingham study. Clin Endocrinol Metab 1976;5(2):367–75.

[57] Haskell WL, Alderman EL, Fair JM, et al. Effects of intensive multiple risk factor reduction on coronary atherosclerosis and clinical cardiac events in men and women with coronary artery disease. The Stanford Coronary Risk Intervention Project (SCRIP). Circulation 1994;89(3):975–90.

[58] Buchwald H, Williams SE, Matts JP, et al. Overall mortality in the program on the surgical control of the hyperlipidemias. J Am Coll Surg 2002;195(3):327–31.

[59] Karason K, Wikstrand J, Sjostrom L, et al. Weight loss and progression of early atherosclerosis in the carotid artery: a four-year controlled study of obese subjects. Int J Obes Relat Metab Disord 1999;23(9):948–56.

[60] Sampalis JS, Sampalis F, Christou N. Impact of bariatric surgery on cardiovascular and musculoskeletal morbidity. Surg Obes Relat Dis 2006;2(6):587–91.

[61] Ramani GV, Mathier MA. Safety and efficacy of bariatric surgery in morbidly obese patients with severe heart failure. J Am Coll Cardiol 2007;49(9):62A–63A.

[62] Papaioannou A, Michaloudis D, Fraidakis O, et al. Effects of weight loss on QT interval in morbidly obese patients. Obes Surg 2003;13:869–73.

[63] Sjostrom L. Soft and hard endpoints over 5 to 18 years in the intervention trial Swedish obese subjects. Obes Rev 2006;7(Suppl 2):27.

[64] Peeters A, O'Brien P, Laurie C, et al. Does weight loss improve survival? Comparison of a bariatric surgical cohort with a community based control group. Obes Rev 2006;7(Suppl 2):95.

[65] Adams T, Gress R, Smith S, et al. Long-term mortality following gastric bypass surgery. Obes Rev 2006;7(Suppl 2):94.

[66] MacMahon SW, Wilcken DE, Macdonald GJ. The effect of weight reduction on left ventricular mass. A randomized controlled trial in young, overweight hypertensive patients. N Engl J Med 1986;314:334–9.

[67] Randall OS, Kwagyan J, Huang X, et al. Effect of diet and exercise on pulse pressure and cardiac function in morbid obesity: analysis of 24 hour ambulatory blood pressure. J Clin Hypertens 2005;7:455–63.

[68] Facchini M, Malfatto G, Sala L, et al. Changes of autonomic cardiac profile after a 3-week integrated body weight reduction program in severely obese patients. J Endocrinol Invest 2003;26:138–42.

[69] Poirier P, Hernandez TL, Weil KM, et al. Impact of diet-induced weight loss on the cardiac autonomic nervous system in severe obesity. Obes Res 2003;11:1040–7.

[70] Alpert MA, Terry BE, Kelly DL. Effect of weight loss on cardiac chamber size, wall thickness and left ventricular function in morbid obesity. Am J Cardiol 1985;55:783–6.

[71] Sugerman HJ, Baron PL, Fairman RP, et al. Hemodynamic dysfunction in obesity hypoventilation syndrome and the effects of treatment with surgically induced weight loss. Ann Surg 1988;207:604–13.

[72] Karason K, Wallentin I, Larsson B, et al. Effects of obesity and weight loss on left ventricular mass and relative wall thickness: survey and intervention study. BMJ 1997;315:912–6.

[73] Karason K, Wallentin I, Larsson B, et al. Effects of obesity and weight loss on cardiac function and valvular performance. Obes Res 1998;6:422–9.

[74] Kanoupakis E, Michaloudis D, Fraidakis O, et al. Left ventricular function and cardiopulmonary performance following surgical treatment of morbid obesity. Obes Surg 2001;11:552–8.

[75] Willens HJ, Chakko SC, Byers P, et al. Effects of weight loss after gastric bypass bypass on right and left ventricular function assessed by tissue Doppler imaging. Am J Cardiol 2005;95:1521–4.

[76] Seres L, Lopez-Ayerbe J, Coll R, et al. Increased exercise capacity after surgically induced weight loss in morbid obesity. Obesity 2006;14:273–9.

[77] Himeno E, Nishino K, Nakashima Y, et al. Weight reduction regresses left ventricular mass regardless of blood pressure level in obese subjects. Am Heart J 1996;131:313–9.

[78] Straznicky NE, Lambert EA, Lambert GW, et al. Effects of dietary weight loss on sympathetic activity and cardiac risk factors associated with the metabolic syndrome. J Clin Endocrinol Metab 2005;90:5998–6005.

[79] van Dielen FM, Buurman WA, Hadfoune M, et al. Macrophage inhibitory factor, plasminogen activator inhibitor-1, other acute phase proteins, and inflammatory mediators

normalize as a result of weight loss in morbidly obese subjects treated with gastric restrictive surgery. J Clin Endocrinol Metab 2004;89:4062–8.

[80] Libby P. Inflammation and cardiovascular disease mechanisms. Am J Clin Nutr 2006;83: 456S–60S.

[81] Kasasbeh E, Chi DS, Krishnaswamy G. Inflammatory aspects of sleep apnea and their cardiovascular consequences. South Med J 2006;99:58–67.

[82] Kotidis EV, Koliakos GG, Baltzopoulos VG, et al. Serum ghrelin, leptin and adiponectin levels before and after weight loss: comparison of three methods of treatment—a prospective study. Obes Surg 2006;16:1425–32.

[83] Friedman JM, Halaas JL. Leptin and the regulation of body weight in mammals. Nature 1998;395:763–70.

[84] Munzberg H, Myers MG. Molecular and anatomical determinants of central leptin resistance. Nat Neurosci 2005;8:566–70.

[85] Purdham DM, Zou MX, Rajapurohitam V, et al. Rat heart is a site of leptin production and action. Am J Physiol Heart Circ Physiol 2004;287:H2877–84.

[86] Wolk R, Deb A, Caplice NM, et al. Leptin receptor and functional effects of leptin in human endothelial progenitor cells. Atherosclerosis 2005;183:131–9.

[87] Meisel SR, Ellis M, Pariente C, et al. Serum leptin levels increase following acute myocardial infarction. Cardiology 2001;95:206–11.

[88] Schulze PC, Kratzsch J, Linke A, et al. Elevated serum levels of leptin and soluble receptor in patients with advanced chronic heart failure. Eur J Heart Fail 2003;5:33–40.

[89] Barouch LA, Berkowitz DE, Harrison RW, et al. Disruption of leptin signaling contributes to cardiac hypertrophy independently of body weight in mice. Circulation 2003;108: 754–9.

[90] Xu FP, Chen MS, Wang YZ, et al. Leptin induces ventricular hypertrophy via endothelin-1-reactive oxygen species pathway in cultured neonatal rat cardiomyocytes. Circulation 2004;110:1269–75.

[91] Perego L, Pizzocri P, Corradi D, et al. Circulating leptin correlates with left ventricular mass in morbid (grade III) obesity before and after weight loss induced by bariatric surgery: a potential role for leptin in mediating human left ventricular hypertrophy. J Clin Endocrinol Metab 2005;90:4087–93.

[92] Wallace AM, McMahon AD, Packard CJ, et al. Plasma leptin and the risk of cardiovascular disease in the west of Scotland coronary prevention study (WOSCOPS). Circulation 2001;104:3052–6.

[93] Piatti P, Di Mario C, Monti LD, et al. Association of insulin resistance hyperleptinemia, and impaired nitric oxide release with in stent restenosis in patients undergoing coronary stenting. Circulation 2003;108:2074–81.

[94] Smith CC, Mocanu MM, Davidson SM, et al. Leptin, the obesity related hormone, exhibits direct cardioprotective effects. Br J Pharmacol 2006;149:5–13.

[95] Greer JJ, Ware DP, Lefer DJ. Myocardial infarction and heart failure in the db/db diabetic mouse. Am J Physiol Heart Circ Physiol 2006;290:H146–53.

[96] Goldstein BJ, Scalia R. Adiponectin: a novel adipokine linking adipocytes and vascular function. J Clin Endocrinol Metab 2004;89:2563–8.

[97] Yamamoto Y, Hirose H, Saito I, et al. Adiponectin, an adipocyte-derived protein, predicts future insulin resistance: two-year follow-up study in Japanese population. J Clin Endocrinol Metab 2004;89:87–90.

[98] Koenig W, Khuseyinova N, Baumert J, et al. Serum concentrations of adiponectin and risk of type 2 diabetes mellitus and coronary heart disease in apparently healthy middle-aged men: results from the 18-year follow-up of a large cohort from southern Germany. J Am Coll Cardiol 2006;48:1369–77.

[99] Pischon T, Girman CJ, Hotamisligil GS, et al. Plasma adiponectin levels and risk of myocardial infarction in men. JAMA 2004;291:1730–7.

[100] Sattar N, Wannamethee G, Sarwar N, et al. Adiponectin and coronary heart disease: a prospective study and meta-analysis. Circulation 2006;114:623–9.
[101] Kistorp C, Faber J, Galatius S, et al. Plasma adiponectin, body mass index, and mortality in patients with chronic heart failure. Circulation 2005;112:1756–62.
[102] Hermann TS, Li W, Dominguez H, et al. Quinapril treatment increases insulin-stimulated endothelial function and adiponectin gene expression in patients with type 2 diabetes. J Clin Endocrinol Metab 2006;91:1001–8.
[103] Swarbrick MM, Austrheim-Smith IT, Stanhope KL, et al. Circulating concentrations of high-molecular-weight adiponectin are increased following Roux-en-Y gastric bypass surgery. Diabetologia 2006;49:2552–8.

THE MEDICAL
CLINICS
OF NORTH AMERICA

ELSEVIER
SAUNDERS

Med Clin N Am 91 (2007) 433–442

Pulmonary Considerations in Obesity and the Bariatric Surgical Patient

Garth Davis, MD[a],*, Jitesh A. Patel, MD[b],
Daniel J. Gagne, MD[c]

[a]Houston Surgical Consultants, 6560 Fannin Street, Suite 738, Houston, TX 77030, USA
[b]Department of Surgery, Allegheny General Hospital, 320 East North Avenue,
Pittsburgh, PA 15212, USA
[c]Minimally Invasive Surgery Program, Department of Surgery, The Western Pennsylvania
Hospital, Temple University, 4727 Friendship Avenue, Suite 140,
Pittsburgh, PA 15224, USA

Severe obesity can be associated with significant alterations in normal cardiopulmonary physiology. The pathophysiologic effects of obesity on a patient's pulmonary function are multiple and complex. The impact of obesity on morbidity and mortality are often underestimated. Bariatric surgery has been shown to be the most effective modality of reliable and durable treatment for severe obesity [1]. Surgical weight loss improves and, in most cases, completely resolves the pulmonary health problems associated with obesity [2].

Pathophysiology of pulmonary dysfunction due to obesity

Obese patients sustain a combination of mechanical and inflammatory mediated insults that result in pulmonary disability. The excess fat externally and internally compresses the thoracic cavity. Evidence suggests that fatty infiltration of the accessory muscles of breathing can decrease compliance of the chest wall. Central adiposity can increase intra-abdominal pressure causing cephalad displacement of the diaphragm. This displacement results in a chronic abdominal compartment syndrome resulting in diminished lung volumes and suboptimal pulmonary dynamics. Obesity also leads to increased pulmonary blood volume which competes for space in the chest cavity, further decreasing lung volumes [3].

---

* Corresponding author.
E-mail address: gpdtx@yahoo.com (G. Davis).

0025-7125/07/$ - see front matter © 2007 Published by Elsevier Inc.
doi:10.1016/j.mcna.2007.02.001
medical.theclinics.com

The result of this mechanical load is dramatic when evaluated by pulmonary function tests. As the body mass index (BMI) increases, the forced expiratory volume at one second (FEV_1), forced vital capacity (FVC), total lung capacity (TLC), expiratory reserve volume (ERV), and functional residual capacity (FRC) are markedly reduced [4–7]. The FRC and ERV are especially affected. When compared with a person with a BMI of 20 kg/m^2, a person with a BMI of 30 kg/m^2 has lost 66% of FRC and 70% of ERV [7]. Possibly an even more important correlate of the impact of obesity on pulmonary function than BMI is the waist-to-hip ratio—a determinant of abdominal adiposity [8].

The large amount of work it takes to move an obese body combined with the decreased compliance of the chest wall can lead to a subjective sensation of dyspnea, commonly seen in obese patients. To make matters worse, evidence suggests that this continued "battle to breathe" can lead to respiratory muscle weakness as evidenced by decreases in maximum inspiratory pressure in a comparison with nonobese subjects [9,10]. For these reasons, it is not hard to understand that, with weak muscles, poor chest wall compliance, and a large body habitus, exercise tolerance is poor in the severely obese patient.

Evidence suggests that mechanical forces are not the only insult of obesity on respiratory function; there are also pathophysiologic changes at the molecular level. Obesity can be characterized as a disease of systemic inflammation. C-reactive protein, tumor necrosis factor, and interleukin-6 can all be elevated in the obese patient and can affect airway reactivity [11]. In addition, leptin, which is produced by adipocytes and thereby elevated in the obese patient, may increase airway reactivity [12].

These pathologic changes caused by obesity from the molecular to the anatomic level result in multiple pulmonary-related comorbidities, including asthma, obstructive sleep apnea (OSA), obesity hypoventilation (OHS), and pulmonary hypertension.

Asthma

Asthma currently affects 5% of the population, and the percentage is increasing yearly [13]. Likewise, we are seeing a worldwide epidemic of obesity with numbers that are increasing at a notable rate. This increase has led some people to postulate that the rise in asthma is secondary to the rise in obesity. An increasing body of literature demonstrates a relationship between obesity and asthma, and these two entities may be causally related [14–18]. In a multivariate prospective analysis of 85,911 nurses, Camargo and colleagues [15] demonstrated that the BMI had a strong, independent, and positive association with the risk for adult onset asthma.

The mechanism whereby obesity leads to asthma is likely multifactorial. The pro-inflammatory state found in obesity probably contributes to airway reactivity. Gastroesophageal reflux disease offers another confounding factor. The high rate of this disease in obese patients secondary to increased intra-abdominal pressure may lead to high esophageal reflux and chronic aspiration creating hypersensitive airways. Interestingly, even the pulmonary mechanics may lead to asthma [19,20]. A study by Wang and colleagues [21] exposed normal weight individuals to external chest and abdominal mass loading, increased chest blood volume by leg compression, and then measured airway responsiveness. An increase in airway sensitivity was found in lean subjects when exposed to forces that might be seen in an obese patient. It has been suggested that sex hormones, although the mechanism is poorly understood, may be a factor in inducing asthma. This relationship is supported by the higher correlation of BMI to asthma in women [22,23].

Obstructive sleep apnea

OSA is the intermittent cessation of breathing during sleep due to the collapse of the pharyngeal airway, resulting in multiple apneic or hypopneic events. During the apneic events, the arterial oxygen pressure (PaO_2) decreases and the partial pressure of carbon dioxide ($PaCO_2$) increases, which causes an increase in ventilatory effort and subsequently triggers arousal. This effect is often accompanied by dysrhythmias, bradycardia, and heart block. Sympathetic tone is likewise increased and contributes to pulmonary and systemic hypertension. This state can ultimately lead to cor pulmonale [24–26]. These symptoms are all reversible with successful treatment of OSA. Polysomnography (PSG) is the gold standard for the diagnosis and assessment of treatment for OSA [25].

OSA is commonly associated with obesity yet is underdiagnosed by physicians in general [27,28]. It is estimated that 12% to 40% of morbidly obese patients have OSA. Despite this high prevalence, these numbers may actually be a substantial underestimate of its true prevalence. In two separate studies, patients presenting for bariatric surgery were consecutively screened for OSA and 71% to 77% met the criteria. In the obese population, there should be a low threshold to evaluate for OSA [29,30].

A simple history and physical examination can provide clues to whether a patient has OSA. Obesity, snoring, snorting or arousal, morning headaches, and daytime sleepiness are all signs and symptoms of OSA. BMI is unreliable in predicting OSA; however, a BMI of 35 kg/m^2 or greater is a risk factor, in addition to a neck circumference greater than 41 cm and male sex. These signs and symptoms should lead physicians to evaluate the patient with PSG.

The obesity hypoventilation syndrome

OHS, also known as pickwickian syndrome, is defined as having a BMI greater than 30 kg/m^2 and an awake $PaCO_2$ greater than 45 mm Hg in the absence of a known cause for hypoventilation. It is frequently accompanied by OSA. Like OSA, OHS is underdiagnosed. Studies have shown that as many as 30% of hospitalized obese patients have OHS [31].

OHS shares much of its pathogenesis with OSA; however, there appears to be an element of decreased ventilatory drive in the presence of an elevated PCO_2 in comparisons with BMI-matched subjects who do not have OHS [32]. There is speculation that leptin insensitivity, also thought to cause obesity, may have an effect on suppressing the ventilatory response [33].

OHS should be suspected in any obese patient with hypoxemia, hypersomnolence, and cor pulmonale. Evaluation should include a complete blood count to evaluate for erythrocytosis, arterial blood gas to evaluate $PaCO_2$, bicarbonate to look for chronic compensatory metabolic alkalosis, and levels of thyroid-stimulating hormone and creatine phosphokinase to look for other possible causes of hypoventilation [34].

Perioperative considerations

Candidates for bariatric surgery should be evaluated for pulmonary health problems related to their obesity. Screening studies such as sleep studies and pulmonary function tests are an important part of the preoperative work-up to avoid perioperative complications. OSA is undiagnosed, and unrecognized OSA may greatly influence perioperative morbidity and mortality. There should be a low threshold for OSA screening with PSG in the obese population before weight-loss surgery [29,30]. Once OSA has been diagnosed, continuous positive airway pressure (CPAP) appears to be appropriate therapy in the obese patient perioperatively. Empiric therapy has been suggested for patients unable to complete PSG before surgery [29]. Pulmonary function tests may also be helpful in predicting pulmonary complications in the immediate postoperative period [35].

Preoperative evaluation of the obese patient likely requires a consultation with an anesthesiologist. Obese patients, particularly those with OSA, typically have neck anatomy that makes intubation difficult, that is, a short thick neck with fatty infiltration of the pharyngeal walls. Failed intubation can occur in as many as 5% of attempted surgeries on patients with OSA [36,37]. To further complicate matters, these patients have a small FRC and desaturate quickly during the induction of anesthesia. Identification of a difficult airway in this population may necessitate awake, rapid sequence, or fiberoptic intubation [38,39]. A multidisciplinary approach is essential for the management of these complex patients with minimal physiologic reserve.

Intraoperatively, premorbid pulmonary dysfunction comes into play in patient management, especially during laparoscopic surgery. The pneumoperitoneum necessary to create a "working space" for the surgeon causes a cephalad pressure on the diaphragm, which, in turn, further interferes with the already diminished chest wall compliance and functional lung volumes. The result is a decrease in arterial oxygenation and increased airway pressures. Furthermore, laparoscopy with carbon dioxide insufflation can lead to further carbon dioxide retention and subsequently requires increased elimination [40,41].

Postoperative respiratory complications can also result from pain management. Centrally acting drugs, including benzodiazepines and narcotics, weaken the pharyngeal dilator muscles. In an obese patient, especially one with OSA/OHS, this may result in collapse of the airway and mimic a sleep apneic event. Opioids in combination with the retention of carbon dioxide can further blunt the ventilatory response [36].

It is crucial that all patients be screened for OSA/OHS preoperatively, and, if diagnosed, that they use CPAP postoperatively. Early ambulation and incentive spirometry are vital in preventing atelectasis from splinting owing to pain at abdominal incisions. Atelectasis will further reduce lung compliance and may result in the development of postoperative pneumonia, which can be seen in 1.9% of post bariatric surgery patients [42]. Laparoscopic procedures are typically associated with less postoperative pain, decreased opioid use, and earlier ambulation when compared with open procedures.

Venous thromboembolism and bariatric surgery

The risk for venous thromboembolism is increased in patients undergoing laparoscopic bariatric procedures, in part, due to increased femoral and iliac vein stasis caused by pneumoperitoneum and the reverse Trendelenburg position. The incidence of postoperative deep vein thrombosis detected by duplex ultrasound in select recent reports is 0% to 2.65% [43–47]. Nguyen and colleagues [48] quantified the hemodynamic effect on femoral vein flow during laparoscopic gastric bypass using duplex ultrasound and determined that femoral vein peak systolic velocity is decreased to 57% of baseline. Sequential compression devices were able to ameliorate this effect by decreasing femoral vein peak systolic flow to 22% of baseline.

The reported incidence of pulmonary embolism is 0.84% to 0.95%. Despite seemingly adequate anticoagulation with heparin or low-molecular-weight heparin, there is a persistent risk for pulmonary embolism. Pulmonary embolism is the leading cause of death following bariatric surgery [47, 49,50]. Unfortunately, most of these emboli are detected following discharge and up to 30 days postoperatively.

The presence of chronic hypoxic syndromes, such as OSA, may further increase the risk of thromboemboli because these conditions cause polycythemia. OHS is also a risk factor for pulmonary embolism. In patients deemed to be at high risk, aggressive prophylaxis with preoperative inferior vena cava filter placement, intraoperative heparin infusion, prolonged postoperative anticoagulation, and postoperative warfarin has been suggested. "High-risk" patients were identified as those with heart failure, a BMI of 50 kg/m^2 or greater, or a history of venous thromboembolism or pelvic surgery

[51,52]. Numerous regimens for venous thromboembolism prophylaxis have been suggested [44,53]. Early ambulation and the use of sequential compression devices are universally encouraged for all patients undergoing general anesthesia and may alone be adequate prophylaxis [46]. A consensus for prophylactic anticoagulation does not exist in this patient population [47].

Outcome on pulmonary function following bariatric surgery

Weight loss has been shown to greatly improve or, in some instances, eradicate obesity-related pulmonary dysfunction. These improvements have also been shown following weight-loss surgery [2,34,54–73]. According to the National Institutes Consensus Development Conference Statement on the surgical treatment of obesity, patients with a BMI of 40 kg/m^2 or greater are candidates for bariatric surgery. Because of the relationship between obesity and pulmonary complications and the reversal of this dysfunction with substantial weight loss, the consensus statement also specifies that patients with type II obesity (BMI of 35–40 kg/m^2) are candidates for bariatric surgery if they also have a high-risk cardiopulmonary comorbidity such as OSA or pickwickian syndrome [1]. It has been suggested in other reports that respiratory insufficiency secondary to obesity be considered an indication for weight-loss surgery [57–59].

The majority of weight loss following bariatric procedures occurs 12 to 18 months postoperatively. Within this interval, there is clear evidence that amelioration or even resolution of pulmonary dysfunction occurs. Lung volumes are significantly improved (FVC, TLC, FRC, FEV_1), PaO_2 and arterial oxygen saturation increase, and $PaCO_2$ decreases [60–63]. Furthermore, there is an improvement in ventilation/perfusion along with a reduction in energy expenditure (work of breathing) following weight loss after bariatric surgery [64].

Improvement in OSA is dramatic after surgical weight loss and has been reported in almost every series of bariatric surgery outcomes. A meta-analysis of the bariatric surgery literature by Buchwald and colleagues [2] reviewed 136 fully extracted studies from 2738 citations. This extensive meta-analysis on the effects of bariatric surgery reported on the outcomes of 22,094 patients. Although this meta-analysis reviewed several bariatric surgical procedures, surgical weight loss resulted in the complete resolution of OSA in 85.7% of patients. Following substantial weight loss, as OSA improves, the requirements for CPAP may also change considerably. The use of auto-titrating devices may facilitate the weaning of patients from CPAP support [57,65].

In a report by Scheuller and Weider [58], weight-loss surgery was performed in obese patients (n = 15) primarily as a means for treatment of severe sleep apnea syndrome. Traditional CPAP was unavailable or not tolerated by this cohort of patients. Postoperatively, there was a significant decrease in the average respiratory disturbance index from 96.9 to 11.3. Mean preoperative oxygen saturation increased from 58.7% to 85.2% postoperatively.

Pulmonary hypertension associated with OHS and OSA is also effectively treated following weight-loss surgery. One year following bariatric surgery, Valencia-Flores and colleagues [66] demonstrated a significant decrease in systolic pulmonary artery pressure in all patients. In another more comprehensive study by Sugerman and colleagues [56], pulmonary artery catheters were inserted preoperatively and then reinserted in patients with pulmonary hypertension (n = 18) 3 to 9 months postoperatively. In this cohort, there was a significant improvement or eradication of pulmonary hypertension and systemic hypertension. Furthermore, there was significant improvement in arterial blood gases and left ventricular function.

Severely obese patients with asthma experience resolution or improvement after surgical weight loss. Studies have shown that asthma severity scores improve by an average of 90% with weight loss to a BMI of 30 kg/m^2 [67]. Brolin [68] reported resolution in 56% and improvement in 40% (n = 25) of asthmatics postoperatively. Other groups have reported similar improvement in asthma after bariatric surgery [61,69–72].

Exercise tolerance has also been shown to improve significantly following bariatric surgery. In study by Maniscalco and colleagues [73], patients (n = 15) were followed up prospectively after laparoscopic gastric banding. One-year following surgery, the dyspnea score was significantly decreased, and the distance walked increased from 475.7 m to 626.3 m.

Summary

Evaluation of the bariatric surgery patient should include a thorough history and physical examination to detect previously undiagnosed obesity-related comorbidities. Pulmonary comorbidities are often underdiagnosed, and there is strong evidence for the screening of patients with PSG. Knowledge of these preoperative conditions can allow the practitioner to safeguard against the common pitfalls that can occur in the perioperative setting. A multidisciplinary approach is optimal in these patients and may require preoperative consultation with a pulmonologist or anesthesiologist. Although patients with obesity-related pulmonary dysfunction certainly are at increased risk for perioperative complications, weight-loss surgery provides alleviation or resolution of these premorbid disease processes. Venous thrombolic disease is the primary source of mortality following bariatric surgery, although its prevalence may be substantially decreased with appropriate prophylaxis. In the setting of a careful, multidisciplinary, perioperative evaluation, weight-loss surgery appears to be invaluable in the treatment of obesity-related pulmonary dysfunction.

References

[1] Hubbard VS, Hall WH. Gastrointestinal surgery for severe obesity. Obes Surg 1991;1(3): 257–65.

[2] Buchwald H, Avidor Y, Braunwald E, et al. Bariatric surgery: a systematic review and meta-analysis. JAMA 2004;292(14):1724–37.

[3] Fadell EJ, Richman AD, Ward WW, et al. Fatty infiltration of the respiratory muscles in the pickwickian syndrome. N Engl J Med 1962;266:861–3.

[4] Lazarus R, Sparrow D, Weiss ST. Effects of obesity and fat distribution on ventilatory function: the normative aging study. Chest 1997;111(4):891–8.

[5] Chinn DJ, Cotes JE, Reed JW. Longitudinal effects of change in body mass on measurements of ventilatory capacity. Thorax 1996;51(7):699–704.

[6] Rubinstein I, Zamel N, DuBarry L, et al. Airflow limitation in morbidly obese, nonsmoking men. Ann Intern Med 1990;112(11):828–32.

[7] Jones RL, Nzekwu MM. The effects of body mass index on lung volumes. Chest 2006;130(3): 827–33.

[8] Ochs-Balcom HM, Grant BJ, Muti P, et al. Pulmonary function and abdominal adiposity in the general population. Chest 2006;129(4):853–62.

[9] Weiner P, Waizman J, Weiner M, et al. Influence of excessive weight after gastroplasty on respiratory muscle performance. Thorax 1988;53(1):39–42.

[10] Chlif M, Keochkerian D, Mourlhon C, et al. Non-invasive assessment of the tension-time index of inspiratory muscles at rest in obese male subjects. Int J Obs (Lond) 2005;29(12): 1478–83.

[11] Fantuzzi G. Adipose tissue, adipokines, and inflammation. J Allergy Clin Immunol 2005; 115(5):911–4.

[12] Maffei M, Halaas J, Ravussin E, et al. Leptin levels in human and rodent: measurement of plasma leptin and ob RNA in obese and weight-reduced subjects. Nat Med 1995;1(11): 1155–61.

[13] Centers for Disease Control and Prevention, asthma in the United States, 1982-1992. MMWR Morb Mortal Wkly Rep 1995;43:952–5.

[14] Shaheen SO, Sterne JA, Montgomery SM, et al. Birth weight, body mass index, and asthma in young adults. Thorax 1999;54:396–402.

[15] Camargo CA Jr, Weiss ST, Zhang S, et al. Prospective study of body mass index, weight change, and risk of adult-onset asthma in women. Arch Intern Med 1999;159(21):2582–8.

[16] Tantisira KG, Weiss ST. Complex interactions in complex traits: obesity and asthma. Thorax 2001;56(Suppl 2):64–73.

[17] Chinn S, Downs SH, Anto JM, et al. Incidence of asthma and net change in symptoms in relation to changes in obesity. Eur Respir J 2006;28(4):763–71.

[18] Beuther DA, Weiss ST, Sutherland ER. Obesity and asthma. Am J Respir Crit Care Med 174(2):112–119.

[19] Kasasbeh A, Kasasbeh E, Krishnaswamy G. Potential mechanisms connecting asthma, esophageal reflux, and obesity/sleep apnea complex: a hypothetical review. Sleep Med Rev 2007;11(1):47–58.

[20] Gunnbjornsdottir MI, Omenaas E, Gislason T, et al. Obesity and nocturnal gastro-oesophageal reflux are related to onset of asthma and respiratory symptoms. Eur Respir J 2004;24(1): 116–21.

[21] Wang LY, Cerny FJ, Kufel TJ, et al. Simulated obesity-related changes in lung volume increases airway responsiveness in lean, non-asthmatic subjects. Chest 2006;130(3): 834–40.

[22] Kim S, Camargo CA Jr. Sex-race differences in the relationship between obesity and asthma: the behavioral risk factor surveillance system, 2000. Ann Epidemiol 2003;13(10):666–73.

[23] Tantisira KG, Weiss ST. The pharmacogenetics of asthma therapy. Curr Drug Targets 2006; 7(12):1697–708.

[24] Rama AN, Tekwani SH, Kushida CA. Sites of obstruction in obstructive sleep apnea. Chest 2002;122(4):1139–47.

[25] Gami AS, Caples SM, Somers VK. Obesity and obstructive sleep apnea. Endocrinol Metab Clin North Am 2003;32(4):869–94.

[26] Phillips CL, Cistulli PA. Obstructive sleep apnea and hypertension: epidemiology, mechanisms and treatment effects. Minerva Med 2006;97(4):299–312.

[27] Strollo PJ Jr, Rogers RM. Obstructive sleep apnea. N Engl J Med 1996;334(2):99–104.

[28] Rosen RC, Rosekind M, Rosevear C, et al. Physician education in sleep and sleep disorders: a national survey of US medical schools. Sleep 1993;16(3):244–54.

[29] Frey WC, Pilcher J. Obstructive sleep-related breathing disorders in patients evaluated for bariatric surgery. Obes Surg 2003;13(5):676–83.

[30] O'Keeffe T, Patterson EJ. Evidence supporting routine polysomnography before bariatric surgery. Obes Surg 2004;14(1):23–6.

[31] Nowbar S, Burkart KM, Gonzales R, et al. Obesity associated hypoventilation in hospitalized patients: prevalence, effects, and outcome. Am J Med 2004;116(1):1–7.

[32] Sampson MG, Grassino A. Neuromechanical properties in obese patients during carbon dioxide rebreathing. Am J Med 1983;75(1):81–90.

[33] O'Donnell CP, Schaub CD, Haines AS, et al. Leptin prevents respiratory depression in obesity. Am J Respir Crit Care Med 1999;159(5 Pt 1):1477–84.

[34] Olson AL, Zwillich C. The obesity hypoventilation syndrome. Am J Med 2005;118:948–56.

[35] Hamoui N, Anthone G, Crookes PF. The value of pulmonary function testing prior to bariatric surgery. Obes Surg 2006;16(12):1570–3.

[36] Benumof JL. Obesity, sleep apnea, the airway, and anesthesia. Curr Opin Anaesthesiol 2004; 17(1):21–30.

[37] Siyam MA, Benhamou D. Difficult endotracheal intubation in patients with sleep apnea syndrome. Anesth Analg 2002;95(4):1098–102.

[38] Ezri T, Muzikant G, Medalion B, et al. Anesthesia for restrictive bariatric surgery (gastric bypass not included): laparoscopic vs open procedures. Int J Obes Relat Metab Disord 2004;28(9):1157–62.

[39] Pellis T, Leykin Y, Albano G, et al. Perioperative management and monitoring of a super-obese patient. Obes Surg 2004;14(10):1423–7.

[40] Meininger D, Zwissler B, Byhahn C, et al. Impact of overweight and pneumoperitoneum on hemodynamics and oxygenation during prolonged laparoscopic surgery. World J Surg 2006; 30(4):520–6.

[41] Nguyen NT, Wolfe BM. The physiologic effects of pneumoperitoneum in the morbidly obese. Ann Surg 2005;241(2):219–26.

[42] Nguyen NT, Silver M, Robinson M, et al. Results of a national audit of bariatric surgery performed at academic centers: a 2004 University Health System Consortium Benchmarking Project. Arch Surg 2006;141(5):445–9.

[43] Prystowsky JB, Morasch MD, Eskandari MK, et al. Prospective analysis of the incidence of deep venous thrombosis in bariatric surgery patients. Surgery 2005;138(4):759–63.

[44] Miller MT, Rovito PF. An approach to venous thromboembolism prophylaxis in laparoscopic Roux-en-Y gastric bypass surgery. Obes Surg 2004;14(6):731–7.

[45] Westling A, Bergqvist D, Bostrom A, et al. Incidence of deep venous thrombosis in patients undergoing obesity surgery. World J Surg 2002;26(4):470–3.

[46] Gonzalez QH, Tishler DS, Plata-Munoz JJ, et al. Incidence of clinically evident deep venous thrombosis after laparoscopic Roux-en-Y gastric bypass. Surg Endosc 2004; 18(7):1082–4.

[47] Wu EC, Barba CA. Current practices in the prophylaxis of venous thromboembolism in bariatric surgery. Obes Surg 2000;10(1):7–13.

[48] Nguyen NT, Cronan M, Braley S, et al. Duplex ultrasound assessment of femoral venous flow during laparoscopic and open gastric bypass. Surg Endosc 2003;17(2):285–90.

[49] Carmody BJ, Sugerman HJ, Kellum JM, et al. Pulmonary embolism complicating bariatric surgery: detailed analysis of a single institution's 24-year experience. J Am Coll Surg 2006; 203(6):831–7.

[50] Hamad GG, Bergqvist D. Venous thromboembolism in bariatric surgery patients: an update of risk and prevention. Surg Obes Relat Dis 2007;3(1):97–102.

[51] Frezza EE, Wachtel MS. A simple venous thromboembolism prophylaxis protocol for patients undergoing bariatric surgery. Obesity (Silver Spring) 2006;14(11):1961–5.

[52] Abou-Nukta F, Alkhoury F, Arroyo K, et al. Clinical pulmonary embolus after gastric bypass surgery. Surg Obes Relat Dis 2006;2(1):24–8.

[53] Cotter SA, Cantrell W, Fisher B, et al. Efficacy of venous thromboembolism prophylaxis in morbidly obese patients undergoing gastric bypass surgery. Obes Surg 2005;15(9):1316–20.

[54] Sugerman HJ, Fairman RP, Baron PL, et al. Gastric surgery for respiratory insufficiency of obesity. Chest 1986;90(1):81–6.

[55] Sugerman HJ, Fairman RP, Sood RK, et al. Long-term effects of gastric surgery for treating respiratory insufficiency of obesity. Am J Clin Nutr 1992;55(2 Suppl):587S–601S.

[56] Sugerman HJ, Baron PL, Fairman RP, et al. Hemodynamic dysfunction in obesity ventilation syndrome and the effects of surgically induced weight loss. Ann Surg 1988;207(5): 604–13.

[57] Boone KA, Cullen JJ, Mason EE, et al. Impact of vertical banded gastroplasty on respiratory insufficiency of severe obesity. Obes Surg 1996;6(6):454–8.

[58] Scheuller M, Weider D. Bariatric surgery for treatment of sleep apnea syndrome in 15 morbidly obese patients: long-term results. Otolaryngol Head Neck Surg 2001;125(4):299–302.

[59] Dixon JB, Schachter LM, O'Brien PE. Polysomnography before and after weight loss in obese patients with severe sleep apnea. Int J Obes (Lond) 2005;29(9):1048–54.

[60] Wadstrom C, Muller-Suur R, Backman L. Influence of excessive weight loss on respiratory function: a study of obese patients following gastroplasty. Eur J Surg 1991;157(5):341–6.

[61] He M, Stubbs R. Gastric bypass surgery for severe obesity: what can be achieved? N Z Med J 2004;117(1207):U1207.

[62] Davila-Cervantes A, Dominguez-Cherit G, Borunda D, et al. Impact of surgically induced weight loss on respiratory function: a prospective analysis. Obes Surg 2004;14(10):1389–92.

[63] Aaron SD, Fergusson D, Dent R, et al. Effect of weight reduction on respiratory function and airway reactivity in obese women. Chest 2004;125(6):2046–52.

[64] Refsum HE, Holter PH, Lovig T, et al. Pulmonary function and energy expenditure after marked weight loss in obese women: observations before and one year after gastric banding. Int J Obes 1990;14(2):175–83.

[65] Lankford DA, Proctor CD, Richard R. Continuous positive airway pressure (CPAP) changes in bariatric surgery patients undergoing rapid weight loss. Obes Surg 2005;15(3): 336–41.

[66] Valencia-Flores M, Orea A, Herrera M, et al. Effect of bariatric surgery on obstructive sleep apnea and hypopnea syndrome, electrocardiogram, and pulmonary arterial pressure. Obes Surg 2004;14(6):755–62.

[67] Ford ES. The epidemiology of obesity and asthma. J Allergy Clin Immunol 2005;115(5): 897–909.

[68] Brolin RE. Results of obesity surgery. Gastroenterol Clin North Am 1987;16(2):317–38.

[69] Dhabuwala A, Cannan RJ, Stubbs RS. Improvement in co-morbidities following weight loss from gastric bypass surgery. Obes Surg 2000;10(5):428–35.

[70] Hall JC, Watts JM, O'Brien PE, et al. Gastric surgery for morbid obesity: the Adelaide study. Ann Surg 1990;211(4):419–27.

[71] Macgregor AM, Greenberg RA. Effect of surgically induced weight loss on asthma in the morbidly obese. Obes Surg 1993;3(1):15–21.

[72] Dixon JB, Chapman L, O'Brien P. Marked improvement in asthma after lap-band surgery for morbid obesity. Obes Surg 1999;9(4):385–9.

[73] Maniscalco M, Zedda A, Giardiello C, et al. Effect of bariatric surgery on the six-minute walk test in severe uncomplicated obesity. Obes Surg 2006;16(7):836–41.

THE MEDICAL
CLINICS
OF NORTH AMERICA

Med Clin N Am 91 (2007) 443–450

Management of Gastrointestinal Disorders in the Bariatric Patient

Troy A. Markel, MD[a], Samer G. Mattar, MD[b],*

[a]Department of Surgery, Indiana University School of Medicine, 545 Barnhill Drive,
EH202, Indianapolis, IN 46202, USA
[b]Clarian Bariatric Center, Department of Surgery, Indiana University School of Medicine,
6625 Network Way, Suite 100, Indianapolis, IN 46278, USA

Morbid obesity continues to grow at an alarming rate. In 2000, approximately 30.5% of the US population was considered obese and 64.5% overweight [1]. As of 2004, 35% of Americans were considered to have a body mass index (BMI) over 30. The greater majority of these individuals have tried numerous weight loss diets with modest, and most often transient results. On the other hand, several studies have highlighted the effectiveness and durability of bariatric surgery, of which Roux-en-Y gastric bypass (RYGBP) is the most popular, in achieving profound weight loss and amelioration, if not resolution, of numerous comorbidities. The popularity of weight loss surgery has been enhanced by the adoption of laparoscopic techniques, thereby catapulting these operations to the forefront of potential solutions for morbid obesity. A phenomenal rise has occurred in the incidence of gastric bypass operations; nearly 140,000 such procedures were performed in 2005.

As the number of patients undergoing RYGBP increases, the patient population presenting to primary care physicians with previous gastric bypass will also increase. Accordingly, it will become imperative for primary care physicians to be familiar and comfortable with the care of these patients. Physicians must not only understand the physiologic, metabolic, and psychologic manifestations of morbid obesity, but also be cognizant of the predicted improvement in comorbidities and the potential complications that patients may face. Most post gastric bypass changes occur within the gastrointestinal tract. Many physicians will be required to treat bariatric patients with liver and biliary disease, as well as gastroesophageal reflux

* Corresponding author.
E-mail address: smattar@iupui.edu (S.G. Mattar).

0025-7125/07/$ - see front matter © 2007 Elsevier Inc. All rights reserved.
doi:10.1016/j.mcna.2007.01.004 *medical.theclinics.com*

disease (GERD) and the metabolic syndrome that are pertinent to this group of patients.

This review focuses on the care of gastrointestinal disorders in postoperative gastric bypass patients. It addresses the more common concerns that patients and their physicians have with regards to the effect of bariatric surgery on gastrointestinal disorders such as GERD and nonalcoholic steatohepatitis (NASH). The literature is reviewed concerning the debate over simultaneous cholecystectomy at the time of bypass for postoperative risk reduction of cholecystitis. The utility of gastric bypass surgery in the cirrhotic patient is also addressed.

Nonalcoholic fatty liver disease

Nonalcoholic fatty liver disease (NAFLD) includes a spectrum of liver disease from steatosis to fibrosis and cirrhosis. NAFLD is estimated to affect 10% to 24% of the population worldwide, 30% to 100% of the adult obese population [2], and approximately 53% of obese children [3]. Obesity is a predictive factor for fibrosis and the progression to NASH and advanced liver disease, with BMI being the only independent predictor of the degree of fat infiltration in the liver [4]. Several studies focusing on liver disease in the bariatric population have demonstrated ultrasonographic evidence of fatty liver in many of the patients studied. Thirty percent of these patients also had histologically documented evidence of NASH [5–8]. Furthermore, the majority of obese patients with NASH who progress to cirrhosis die of the complications associated with their liver disease [9,10].

Weight loss surgery results in dramatic weight loss and is a favorable treatment option for NASH in the bariatric population. Several studies have demonstrated that patients with NASH who undergo bariatric weight loss surgery have improvement in their liver disease [11–13]. In a 2006 study by de Almeida and colleagues [13], 16 patients underwent liver biopsy at the time of RYGBP and then again at designated follow-up. All of the patients exhibited signs of gross and histologic NASH at the time of initial biopsy. A follow-up biopsy approximately 2 years later showed complete regression of disease in 93% of the patients and marked improvement in the one patient who had incomplete regression.

The authors' work supports de Almeida's study. We analyzed data from 70 patients over a 5-year period who had agreed to undergo postoperative liver biopsy. Liver steatosis improved from 88% preoperatively to 8% at the postoperative biopsy approximately 15 months after RYGBP. Furthermore, fibrosis, inflammation, and the metabolic syndrome associated with obesity were dramatically improved [12]. In addition, variables such as lipid and triglyceride profiles, as well as glucose and hemoglobin A_{1C} levels, were dramatically improved after surgery [14].

Laparoscopic gastric band placement also seems to be an effective therapeutic option for NASH. Thirty-six obese patients underwent laparoscopic gastric banding and simultaneous liver biopsy. At a mean 2-year follow-up, a repeat liver biopsy was obtained. Major improvements in lobular steatosis, necroinflammatory changes, and fibrosis were noted at the time of the second biopsy. Portal tract abnormalities remained unchanged; however, 32 of the patients demonstrated complete regression of NASH [15].

It would seem beneficial to refer patients earlier in the course of obesity for RYGBP, with the aim of preventing NASH or arresting or reversing the progression to advanced liver disease in patients who carry the diagnosis of fatty liver. Even patients with advanced liver disease may benefit. A 2005 study by Cobb and colleagues [16] demonstrated that laparoscopic surgical procedures, including RYGBP, were safe in patients with mild to moderately advanced liver disease. An additional study by Dallal and colleagues [17] reviewed their experience with 30 cirrhotic patients undergoing laparoscopic RYGBP. The minor complication rate was 30% with no related postoperative deaths. The patients in this study tended to be male, older, and had a higher incidence of diabetes and hypertension. Although the study did not stratify data based on Child's class of liver disease, laparoscopic RYGBP was safe in patients with mild-to-moderate cirrhosis and liver failure.

Severe liver disease also does not preclude patients from undergoing gastric bypass. There are several accounts in the literature with favorable outcomes in which orthotopic liver transplant patients at a later time underwent laparoscopic gastric bypass for treatment of recurrent steatohepatitis and metabolic syndrome [18,19].

Laparoscopic banding and RYGBP are effective therapies for morbidly obese patients with NASH or mild to moderately advanced liver diseases. Although advanced liver disease increases the morbidity of the surgical weight loss procedure, gastric bypass can be achieved successfully in well-prepared patients.

Cholecystitis/cholecystectomy

Obesity constitutes a clear risk factor for cholecystitis. As patients rapidly lose weight, the bile acids tend to precipitate within the gallbladder, leading to the increased incidence of stones. As such, a strong debate exists as to whether simultaneous cholecystectomy should be performed at the time of gastric bypass. Some argue that cholecystectomy should be performed routinely [20], whereas others favor preoperative ultrasound evaluation of the gallbladder and cholecystectomy only if stones are present [21]. Still others contend that the obese population should be treated like the nonobese, and that cholecystectomy should only be performed for symptomatic stones [22,23].

Certain studies have demonstrated increased gallbladder disease in obese patients, including gallstones, polyps, cholesterolosis, and chronic cholecystitis [23]. Indeed, more than 80% of obese patients exhibit one of these lesions, with gallstones being the most common finding. Many patients remain asymptomatic, resulting in the basis for the controversies at hand.

In one retrospective study of more than 500 patients over a 5.5-year period, approximately 15% of patients were found to have gallstones at the time of gastric bypass. These patients underwent simultaneous cholecystectomy. Only 3% of patients required cholecystectomy after gastric bypass for symptomatic cholecystitis. An additional study by Taylor and colleagues [24] supports these data. Their study found that only 14% of patients required post gastric bypass cholecystectomy, whereas approximately 24% had concomitant or prior cholecystectomy. Furthermore, they found no increased biliary duct injury if cholecystectomy was postponed until needed [22]. In a third prospective study, it was shown that as many as 92% of prophylactic cholecystectomies would have been performed unnecessarily [25]; therefore, it appears that most of the gallstones formed after weight loss surgeries are asymptomatic. The authors conclude that prophylactic cholecystectomy is not warranted at the time of weight loss surgery.

Even patients carrying gallstones on presentation for gastric bypass may be spared an unnecessary cholecystectomy. A recent study showed that 34 of 104 patients had positive preoperative ultrasound findings. Of these, 20 patients were symptomatic and received cholecystectomy, whereas 12 exhibited no signs of cholecystitis and were treated expectantly. At a mean follow-up of 26 months, only 1 of the 12 patients required cholecystectomy [26] for symptomatic disease. These findings question the role of routine ultrasound interrogation of the gallbladder in asymptomatic preoperative patients presenting for weight loss surgery.

Medical prophylaxis, such as the postoperative administration of ursodeoxycholic acid (ursodiol), is used by many surgeons to reduce the risk of gallstone formation after weight loss surgery. Rapid weight loss may promote precipitation of cholesterol in the gallbladder, and ursodiol prevents excess bile absorption and cholesterol precipitation. One study supports this approach, demonstrating that 72% of patients who were prescribed the drug postoperatively and who underwent an ultrasound at 10 months were gallstone free [27]. This study did not have a control; therefore, one cannot adequately conclude that ursodiol was the reason for the lack of visualized stones. The study by Papasavas and coworkers [26] did not provide postoperative ursodiol therapy. The findings suggested that the number of cholecystectomies would have to be reduced by 70% for the drug to have a therapeutic effect.

One of the strongest studies using ursodiol was a 2003 randomized double-blind controlled trial in which 41 patients were randomly assigned to receive ursodiol, ibuprofen, or a placebo after gastric bypass. Patients continued the drug for 6 months postoperatively. At 12-month follow-up,

71% of the patients had gallstones, of which 41% were symptomatic. This study demonstrated that not only were obese patients prone to gallstones but also that ursodiol was not efficacious in preventing stone formation [28]. Because the drug is associated with side effects in more than 25% of patients, lack of compliance may have been an issue in this study.

Based on the information presented herein, physicians can use the same criteria for cholecystectomy in the morbidly obese population as in the general population. In addition, it appears that the use of postoperative medications such as ursodiol is not only costly but also may lack efficacy. Physicians should treat gallstones in the obese population only when symptomatic.

Gastroesophageal reflux disease

Morbid obesity increases the risk for many other health problems, including asthma, sleep apnea, pulmonary hypertension, and GERD. Worldwide, many studies have looked at obesity and its relation to GERD. A recent meta-analysis reviewed 20 studies that included over 18,000 obese patients. Several studies within this meta-analysis demonstrated a strong association between increasing BMI and GERD [29]. Furthermore, there appears to be an increased prevalence of asthma with obesity, and several of the asthma medications used for bronchodilation tend to exacerbate GERD by causing relaxation of the lower esophageal sphincter [30].

RYGBP has been deemed to be a beneficial surgical treatment for GERD in the obese population. Acid, if any, is produced in small quantities within the 15-mL capacity of the gastric pouch. By virtue of gastric exclusion, duodeno-gastro-esophageal reflux is impossible, making RYGBP an ideal surgical means of correcting acid and biliary reflux in the bariatric population. Furthermore, a 2006 study by Csendes and colleagues [31] demonstrated a 2.1% incidence of Barrett's esophagitis in an obese population of 557 undergoing RYGBP. Three of these patients had intestinal metaplasia of the cardia. Postoperatively, symptoms of reflux were absent in all patients, and signs of erosive esophagitis and peptic ulcer disease were no longer present. Additionally, regression of disease was noted in the patients who had preoperative evidence of intestinal metaplasia.

Other studies have corroborated the work of Csendes. A prospective study that analyzed 606 patients found symptoms of GERD in 239 of the patients. Postoperatively, GERD symptoms decreased in 89% of the patients at 3 months, and 94% reported improvement at the 9-month follow-up. Furthermore, use of medication to treat GERD symptoms decreased by 25% over 9 months [32]. Studies still need to be performed to assess long-term improvement in gastroesophageal reflux symptoms after weight loss surgery.

Some obese patients present for weight loss surgery having previously undergone anti-reflux procedures such as gastric fundoplication. Several investigators have reported their experience with gastric bypass following anti-reflux procedures and have found that, although technically more challenging and carrying a higher risk of morbidity, RYGBP is a feasible method for treating obesity and recurrent symptoms of reflux [33].

Despite being considered the most favorable option for the treatment of GERD in the morbidly obese population, weight loss surgery does not provide uniformly successful results. For reasons that remain unclear, some patients continue to sustain symptoms of GERD after weight loss surgery. In a study by the authors' group that reviewed 369 post-RYGBP patients, seven patients who experienced persistent GERD symptoms that were refractory to high-dose anti-secretory medication and who were objectively proven to have GERD underwent the Stretta procedure. Post procedure, greater than 70% of these patients had relief of reflux symptoms, validating the procedure as an appropriate surgical treatment for recurrent GERD in RYGBP patients [34]. Briefly, the Stretta procedure is an endoluminal technique that involves passing an endoscope into the gastric pouch. Radiofrequency energy is then used to create thermal lesions at the lower esophageal sphincter. These lesions scar, creating increased tissue constriction and thickened muscle in the area of the lower esophageal sphincter. This scar effectively tightens the lower esophageal sphincter and augments the physiologic barrier that prevents reflux of acidic contents.

Another option for the correction of obesity and GERD symptoms is the laparoscopic adjustable band procedure. This procedure entails placing a double-chambered silicone band around the superior portion of the stomach, just distal to the gastroesophageal junction. A 2005 study by Spivak and colleagues [35] examined 163 patients with obesity-related comorbidities. The mean excess percent weight loss was 47%. In addition, 87% of patients noted decreased symptoms of GERD after gastric banding at a mean follow-up of 20 months.

Despite the proposed benefit of banding on reflux in the study by Spivak, multiple other studies have shown worsening reflux symptoms after laparoscopic gastric banding. One particular study used pH probes and esophageal manometry as well as patient symptoms and noted that the prevalence of reflux symptoms and esophagitis was no different after banding when compared with before the procedure. Furthermore, there was an increased trend toward more postoperative esophageal motility disorders [36]. A long-term study examining patients 5 years after gastric banding noted that, although a significant weight loss was achieved, the reoperation rate was increased, and the incidence of postoperative reflux and esophagitis was as high as 44% [37].

Another study showed no change in esophageal motility at 6 months postoperatively but did note that gastric reflux symptoms were improved in the short term. Despite this early resolution of symptoms, most patients had a return of reflux symptoms by 6 months, indicating that RYGBP, and not laparoscopic adjustable gastric banding, may be the procedure of choice for bariatric patients desiring a weight loss surgery for obesity and GERD [38].

Summary

Obesity continues to be a health care problem of global proportion, particularly in view of the numerous chronic comorbidities that eventually shorten life expectancy. Many physicians counsel their patients to lose weight through dieting and exercise. In most cases, these methods are unsuccessful, rendering weight loss surgery the most valid option for morbidly obese patients. Although most patients do well postoperatively, some continue to have gastrointestinal problems and may present to their primary care physician. It is the authors' hope that the information provided herein will aid the primary care physician in the treatment of gastrointestinal disorders occurring in the preoperative and postoperative bariatric patient, providing information on which to base treatment or a referral to a bariatric surgeon.

References

[1] Flegal KM, Carroll MD, Ogden CL, et al. Prevalence and trends in obesity among US adults, 1999-2000. JAMA 2002;288:1723–7.

[2] Luyckx FH, Desaive C, Thiry A, et al. Liver abnormalities in severely obese subjects: effect of drastic weight loss after gastroplasty. Int J Obes Relat Metab Disord 1998;22:222–6.

[3] Franzese A, Vajro P, Argenziano A, et al. Liver involvement in obese children: ultrasonography and liver enzyme levels at diagnosis and during follow-up in an Italian population. Dig Dis Sci 1997;42:1428–32.

[4] Angulo P, Keach JC, Batts KP, et al. Independent predictors of liver fibrosis in patients with nonalcoholic steatohepatitis. Hepatology 1999;30:1356–62.

[5] Sabir N, Sermez Y, Kazil S, et al. Correlation of abdominal fat accumulation and liver steatosis: importance of ultrasonographic and anthropometric measurements. Eur J Ultrasound 2001;14:121–8.

[6] Scheen AJ, Luyckx FH. Obesity and liver disease. Best Pract Res Clin Endocrinol Metab 2002;16:703–16.

[7] Bellentani S, Saccoccio G, Masutti F, et al. Prevalence of and risk factors for hepatic steatosis in Northern Italy. Ann Intern Med 2000;132:112–7.

[8] Yu AS, Keeffe EB. Nonalcoholic fatty liver disease. Rev Gastroenterol Disord 2002;2:11–9.

[9] Hui JM, Kench JG, Chitturi S, et al. Long-term outcomes of cirrhosis in nonalcoholic steatohepatitis compared with hepatitis C. Hepatology 2003;38:420–7.

[10] Ratziu V, Bonyhay L, Di Martino V, et al. Survival, liver failure, and hepatocellular carcinoma in obesity-related cryptogenic cirrhosis. Hepatology 2002;35:1485–93.

[11] Mottin CC, Moretto M, Padoin AV, et al. Histological behavior of hepatic steatosis in morbidly obese patients after weight loss induced by bariatric surgery. Obes Surg 2005;15:788–93.

[12] Mattar SG, Velcu LM, Rabinovitz M, et al. Surgically induced weight loss significantly improves nonalcoholic fatty liver disease and the metabolic syndrome. Ann Surg 2005;242:610–7 [discussion: 618–20].

[13] de Almeida SR, Rocha PR, Sanches MD, et al. Roux-en-Y gastric bypass improves the nonalcoholic steatohepatitis (NASH) of morbid obesity. Obes Surg 2006;16:270–8.

[14] Barker KB, Palekar NA, Bowers SP, et al. Nonalcoholic steatohepatitis: effect of Roux-en-Y gastric bypass surgery. Am J Gastroenterol 2006;101:368–73.

[15] Dixon JB, Bhathal PS, Hughes NR, et al. Nonalcoholic fatty liver disease: improvement in liver histological analysis with weight loss. Hepatology 2004;39:1647–54.

[16] Cobb WS, Heniford BT, Burns JM, et al. Cirrhosis is not a contraindication to laparoscopic surgery. Surg Endosc 2005;19:418–23.

[17] Dallal RM, Mattar SG, Lord JL, et al. Results of laparoscopic gastric bypass in patients with cirrhosis. Obes Surg 2004;14:47–53.

[18] Tichansky DS, Madan AK. Laparoscopic Roux-en-Y gastric bypass is safe and feasible after orthotopic liver transplantation. Obes Surg 2005;15:1481–6.

[19] Duchini A, Brunson ME. Roux-en-Y gastric bypass for recurrent nonalcoholic steatohepatitis in liver transplant recipients with morbid obesity. Transplantation 2001;72:156–9.

[20] Guadalajara H, Sanz Baro R, Pascual I, et al. Is prophylactic cholecystectomy useful in obese patients undergoing gastric bypass? Obes Surg 2006;16:883–5.

[21] Vanek VW, Catania M, Triveri K, et al. Retrospective review of the preoperative biliary and gastrointestinal evaluation for gastric bypass surgery. Surg Obes Relat Dis 2006;2:17–22 [discussion: 22–3].

[22] Swartz DE, Felix EL. Elective cholecystectomy after Roux-en-Y gastric bypass: why should asymptomatic gallstones be treated differently in morbidly obese patients? Surg Obes Relat Dis 2005;1:555–60.

[23] Liem RK, Niloff PH. Prophylactic cholecystectomy with open gastric bypass operation. Obes Surg 2004;14:763–5.

[24] Taylor J, Leitman IM, Horowitz M. Is routine cholecystectomy necessary at the time of Roux-en-Y gastric bypass? Obes Surg 2006;16:759–61.

[25] Caruana JA, McCabe MN, Smith AD, et al. Incidence of symptomatic gallstones after gastric bypass: is prophylactic treatment really necessary? Surg Obes Relat Dis 2005;1:564–7 [discussion: 567–8].

[26] Papasavas PK, Gagne DJ, Ceppa FA, et al. Routine gallbladder screening not necessary in patients undergoing laparoscopic Roux-en-Y gastric bypass. Surg Obes Relat Dis 2006;2:41–6 [discussion: 46–7].

[27] Scott DJ, Villegas L, Sims TL, et al. Intraoperative ultrasound and prophylactic ursodiol for gallstone prevention following laparoscopic gastric bypass. Surg Endosc 2003;17:1796–802.

[28] Wudel LJ Jr, Wright JK, Debelak JP, et al. Prevention of gallstone formation in morbidly obese patients undergoing rapid weight loss: results of a randomized controlled pilot study. J Surg Res 2002;102:50–6.

[29] Corley DA, Kubo A. Body mass index and gastroesophageal reflux disease: a systematic review and meta-analysis. Am J Gastroenterol 2006;101(11):2619–28.

[30] Kostikas K, Papaioannou AI, Gourgoulianis KI. BMI and gastroesophageal reflux in women. N Engl J Med 2006;355:848 [author reply: 849–50].

[31] Csendes A, Burgos AM, Smok G, et al. Effect of gastric bypass on Barrett's esophagus and intestinal metaplasia of the cardia in patients with morbid obesity. J Gastrointest Surg 2006;10:259–64.

[32] Nelson LG, Gonzalez R, Haines K, et al. Amelioration of gastroesophageal reflux symptoms following Roux-en-Y gastric bypass for clinically significant obesity. Am Surg 2005;71:950–3 [discussion: 953–4].

[33] Raftopoulos I, Awais O, Courcoulas AP, et al. Laparoscopic gastric bypass after antireflux surgery for the treatment of gastroesophageal reflux in morbidly obese patients: initial experience. Obes Surg 2004;14:1373–80.

[34] Mattar SG, Qureshi F, Taylor D, et al. Treatment of refractory gastroesophageal reflux disease with radiofrequency energy (Stretta) in patients after Roux-en-Y gastric bypass. Surg Endosc 2006;20:850–4.

[35] Spivak H, Hewitt MF, Onn A, et al. Weight loss and improvement of obesity-related illness in 500 US patients following laparoscopic adjustable gastric banding procedure. Am J Surg 2005;189:27–32.

[36] Suter M, Dorta G, Giusti V, et al. Gastric banding interferes with esophageal motility and gastroesophageal reflux. Arch Surg 2005;140:639–43.

[37] Gutschow CA, Collet P, Prenzel K, et al. Long-term results and gastroesophageal reflux in a series of laparoscopic adjustable gastric banding. J Gastrointest Surg 2005;9:941–8.

[38] de Jong JR, van Ramshorst B, Timmer R, et al. Effect of laparoscopic gastric banding on esophageal motility. Obes Surg 2006;16:52–8.

ELSEVIER
SAUNDERS

Med Clin N Am 91 (2007) 451–469

THE MEDICAL
CLINICS
OF NORTH AMERICA

Psychosocial and Behavioral Status of Patients Undergoing Bariatric Surgery: What to Expect Before and After Surgery

Thomas A. Wadden, PhD[a],*, David B. Sarwer, PhD[a,b],
Anthony N. Fabricatore, PhD[a], LaShanda Jones, PhD[a],
Rebecca Stack, BA[a], Noel S. Williams, MD[b]

[a]Department of Psychiatry, University of Pennsylvania School of Medicine,
3535 Market Street, 3rd Floor, Philadelphia, PA 19104, USA
[b]Department of Surgery, Hospital of the University of Pennsylvania,
34th and Spruce Streets, Philadelphia, PA 19104, USA

Extreme obesity, characterized by a body mass index (BMI) of 40 kg/m^2 or greater, is associated with significantly increased mortality, principally from cardiovascular disease, type 2 diabetes, and several cancers [1,2]. It also is associated with an increased risk of psychosocial complications, including depression, eating disorders, and impaired quality of life [3–5]. This article briefly examines the psychosocial status of extremely obese individuals who seek bariatric surgery and describes changes in functioning that can be expected with surgically induced weight loss. The article combines a review of the literature with clinical impressions gained from the more than 2500 candidates for bariatric surgery whom we have evaluated at the Hospital of the University of Pennsylvania.

Mood and anxiety disorders

Psychiatric status varies greatly among persons who seek bariatric surgery [3–7]. A majority have essentially normal psychosocial functioning; however, approximately 25% to 30% of patients report clinically significant

This article was supported by NIH grants K24-DK065018, R01-DK072452, K23-DK070777, and R01-DK069652.

* Corresponding author. University of Pennsylvania, Center for Weight and Eating Disorders, 3535 Market Street, Suite 3029, Philadelphia, PA 19104.

E-mail address: wadden@mail.med.upenn.edu (T.A. Wadden).

doi:10.1016/j.mcna.2007.01.003　　　　　　　　　*medical.theclinics.com*

symptoms of depression at the time of evaluation for surgery [3,5,8]. Studies that have used a structured, clinical interview have found that about 50% of candidates report a lifetime history of mood disorders (including major depression or dysthymia) or of anxiety disorders (including generalized anxiety disorder or social phobia) [3–7].

Methodologic limitations, including the absence of well defined control groups and the use of suboptimal psychometric measures, prevent definitive interpretation of the rates of psychopathology observed in bariatric surgery candidates. Patients encountered in medical and surgical clinics generally report higher rates of depression and anxiety than persons in the general population [9], potentially because of the emotional distress associated with the physical complications that lead patients to seek medical attention. A recent population study of nearly 40,000 individuals found that persons who had a BMI of 40 kg/m^2 or higher were nearly five times more likely to have experienced an episode of major depression in the past year than were individuals of average weight [10]. This finding strongly suggests that extremely obese individuals are more vulnerable to depression, although the factors responsible for this susceptibility are not clear. Contributors may include the weight-related prejudice and discrimination to which severely obese individuals are subjected [11,12] and the presence of bodily pain [13]. Binge eating disorder (BED) is also associated with increased depression [3,5,8,14,15].

Management of psychiatric complications before surgery

Preoperative depression levels and other forms of psychopathology do not consistently predict weight loss after bariatric surgery [3,5]. Investigators originally expected that psychopathology would be associated with suboptimal weight loss, but some studies found greater weight loss in patients who had depression or a history of psychiatric treatment [16–19]. In summarizing the literature, Herpertz and colleagues [16] concluded that negative affect that is related to patients' distress about their obesity may facilitate weight loss after surgery. By contrast, major depression or other psychopathology, which occurs independent of body weight, may be associated with suboptimal outcomes, including medical complications. This hypothesis merits further study.

The finding that preoperative psychiatric status does not consistently predict weight loss has led some to question the need for a psychosocial evaluation [20]. We believe that such assessment is imperative given the frequent occurrence of clinically significant depression (and other disorders) that requires behavioral or pharmacologic intervention to relieve the patient's suffering. Thorough preoperative care should include the treatment of depression. Practitioners are advised, at a minimum, to screen for depression by using a brief interview [8,21,22] or a paper-and-pencil questionnaire such as the Beck Depression Inventory [23]. Candidates for bariatric surgery should be assessed by a mental health professional who has expertise in obesity and is a member of the perioperative team [24]. Although weight loss generally improves mood, it is not a primary treatment for major depression or other psychiatric conditions [16,21]. Thus, psychiatric care should not be delayed in expectation that weight loss will resolve significant mental health problems [16].

Changes in mood and anxiety after bariatric surgery

The Swedish Obese Subjects (SOS) study provides the best evaluation of changes in mood and anxiety after bariatric surgery [25]. This trial included a carefully matched control group that received traditional diet and exercise counseling. Depression scores fell significantly more at 1 year in surgically treated than in control patients (40% versus 10% reductions, respectively). Similar improvements were observed in anxiety (Fig. 1). At 2 years, mean weight loss, which was induced primarily by vertical banded gastroplasty, was approximately 23% of initial weight. At this time and at a 4-year follow-up evaluation, mood and anxiety levels tended to increase slightly from their 1-year levels [25,26]. Larger weight losses at both times were associated with greater improvements in depression and anxiety [25,26]. Dixon and colleagues [27] reported similar improvements in depression after a 20% reduction in initial weight achieved with laparoscopic adjustable banding.

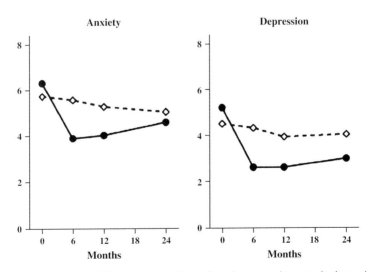

Fig. 1. Participants in the SOS study reported significantly greater decreases in depression and anxiety in the year after surgery than control subjects (*circle*, surgery patients; *square*, control subjects). (*From* Karlsson J, Sjostrom L, Sullivan M. Swedish obese subjects (SOS): an intervention study of obesity. Two-year-follow-up of health-related quality of life (HRQL) and eating behavior after gastric surgery for severe obesity. Int J Obes Relat Metab Disord 1998;22:113–26; with permission.)

The mean presurgical score of 17.7 on the Beck Depression Inventory indicated mild symptoms of depression. One year after surgery, this value fell to 7.8 and remained at 9.0 at 3-year follow-up. These values indicate minimal symptoms of depression.

Risk of suicide in persons who have extreme obesity

The positive findings from these two well conducted studies confirm results from several, smaller uncontrolled investigations (summarized in Refs. [3–6]). Although these findings indicate that bariatric surgery is unlikely to be associated with adverse psychosocial consequences, studies typically have reported only group outcomes and not changes in individual patients. Persons who, before surgery, have a chronic history of major depression or dysthymia may continue to have these problems after surgically induced weight loss [16], despite the favorable changes in mean (ie, group) scores. Moreover, case reports have suggested that patients undergoing bariatric surgery may have a higher-than-expected rate of suicide [28–31]. Factors responsible for this potentially increased risk are not well understood but likely are associated with the emotional burden of extreme obesity [3–5,10,11]. Dong and colleagues [32] recently reported that the risk of attempted suicide in persons who had a BMI of 40 to 49.9 kg/m^2 was 87% greater than that in persons in the general population; a BMI of 50 kg/m^2 or higher was associated with a 122% increased risk. Individuals studied by Dong and colleagues were not candidates for bariatric surgery, thus suggesting that extreme obesity, rather than weight loss surgery alone, increases the risk of suicide. Two other population studies have reported similar findings [10,33]. A case report by Omalu and colleagues [34] suggested that a history of major depression may increase the risk of suicide in persons who undergo bariatric surgery. Each of three individuals who took their lives had a history of severe depression before surgery that persisted postoperatively despite their maintaining losses of 25% to 41% of initial weight at the time of death (which occurred 12–27 months after surgery). These findings underscore the importance of ensuring that patients who have psychiatric disorders receive appropriate mental health care before and after bariatric surgery. More research is needed on the relationships among extreme obesity, depression, surgically induced weight loss, and suicidal behavior.

Eating disorders

Binge eating disorder

Eating disorders are common in patients undergoing bariatric surgery [3–5]. Approximately 10% to 25% of patients suffer from BED, which is characterized by the consumption of an objectively large amount of food in a brief period (<2 hours), during which the individual experiences subjective loss of control [35–39]. Binge episodes cause significant emotional distress. They are not followed by purging (eg, vomiting), which distinguishes BED from bulimia nervosa [35,39]. The presence of BED is associated with increased symptoms of depression, with mean scores for binge eaters falling in the mild to moderate range on the Beck Depression Inventory [3–5,8,14], compared with minimal symptoms of depression for comparably obese individuals without BED. Table 1 summarizes the results of five studies that found that approximately 50% of patients who had BED reported a lifetime history of major depression [14,15,40–43]. Personality disorders, including borderline and narcissistic personality disorder, were common.

Patients tend to over-report the presence of BED. The administration of a semistructured interview results in lower prevalence rates (ie, 5–15%) than does the use of paper-and-pencil questionnaires (ie, estimates as high as 50%) [44]. Thus, patients should be interviewed to confirm that they eat a large amount of food and experience loss of control. Criteria for BED are shown in Box 1.

Night eating syndrome

Approximately 5% to 20% of bariatric surgery candidates also meet criteria for the night eating syndrome (NES) [44–46], which is characterized by the consumption of 35% or more of daily calories after the evening meal [14,47,48]. Patients report frequent nocturnal awakenings, at which time they snack as a means of returning to sleep. This syndrome, like BED, is associated with increased symptoms of depression. NES may be diagnosed using criteria proposed by Allison and Stunkard [14,44].

Table 1
Percentage of BED patients with lifetime comorbidity of DSM diagnoses, as assessed by SCID

Study	Major depression	Any substance abuse or dependence	Any anxiety disorder	Any axis I disorder	Personality disorder
Yanovski et al., 1993	51	12		60	35
Specker et al., 1994	47	72	11.6	72.1	33
Mussel et al., 1996	47	23	18.8	70	
Telch & Stice, 1998	49	9		59	20
Wilfley et al., 2002				63	31

Reprinted from Allison KC, Stunkard AJ. Obesity and eating disorders. Psychiatr Clin North Am 2005;28:55–67.

Box 1. Proposed diagnostic criteria for binge eating disorder

Episodes of binge eating are recurrent and are characterized by the following:

Eating, during a discrete period of time (eg, within any 2-hour period), a quantity of food that is definitely larger than most people would eat during a similar period of time under similar circumstances

A sense of lack of control during the episodes (ie, a feeling that one cannot stop eating or control what or how much one is eating)

Episodes of binge eating are associated with at least three of the following behavioral indicators of loss of control:

Eating much more rapidly than usual

Eating until feeling uncomfortably full

Eating large amounts of food when not feeling physically hungry

Eating alone because of being embarrassed by how much one is consuming

Feeling disgusted with oneself, depressed, or very guilty after overeating

Person feels marked distress regarding binge eating.

Binge eating occurs, on average at least 2 d/wk over a 6-month period.

Binge eating is not associated with regular use of inappropriate compensatory behaviors (eg, purging, fasting, or excessive exercise) and does not occur exclusively during the course of anorexia nervosa or bulimia nervosa.

Effect of eating disorders on postoperative weight loss

Several studies have suggested that the presence of BED before surgery is associated with suboptimal weight loss [5,16,49,50], potentially because of poor adherence to the postoperative diet. In addition, binge eating, whether present preoperatively or not, has been observed in patients who regained weight after achievement of their maximal weight loss with surgery, typically at 18 months [51,52]. These findings, however, have been contradicted by at least four studies that found no differences in weight loss between patients with and without BED [46,53–55]. In addition, all of these studies had methodologic limitations that included small sample sizes, short follow-up assessments, or the retrospective assessment of preoperative binge status [3,5]. Given the absence of definitive data, surgeons and mental health professionals are uncertain whether patients who have BED should be referred for treatment of binge eating before undergoing surgery or should proceed directly to surgery [21,24,56].

Effects of bariatric surgery on binge eating and appetite

Although the presence of BED may limit weight loss after bariatric surgery, the gastric bypass procedure (GBP) may, nonetheless, improve eating-disordered behavior and appetite. In two studies by Hsu and colleagues [49,50], no patients who had BED before surgery reported binge eating postoperatively. Their small pouch size prevented them from consuming objectively large amounts of food. The cessation of binge eating has been reported by others [16,46,57]. Approximately 20% of patients reported subjective binge episodes in which they experienced subjective loss of control of food intake, despite not eating a large amount [49,50]. Such episodes may be associated with smaller weight loss, as suggested by Kalarchian and colleagues [57]. Further study of this issue is needed.

Appetite control

GBP induces weight loss primarily by mechanical restriction of food intake. Patients initially can eat only 1 to 2 oz of food at a sitting because of their small pouch size. They report feeling full more quickly (ie, satiation) and experiencing less hunger (ie, the desire to initiate eating) [25,58]. Reduced hunger after GBP seems to be related to decreased levels of ghrelin, an orexigenic hormone that is secreted primarily by the stomach and acts on hypothalamic neurons (ie, neuropeptide Y and agouti-related protein) that are potent stimulators of food intake [59,60]. As reported by Cummings and colleagues [59], "plasma ghrelin levels rise shortly before and fall shortly after each meal, a pattern that is consistent with a role in the urge to eat." These investigators demonstrated that weight loss after GBP was associated with marked reductions in plasma ghrelin rather than with the increase in this peptide observed after weight loss by diet and exercise. These findings led Cummings and colleagues [59] to conclude that gastric surgery is associated with decreased levels of circulating ghrelin and, thus, the reductions in postoperative hunger. GBP also may increase levels of GLP1 and PYY, each of which inhibits food intake [61]. Thus, GBP seems to induce weight loss, in part, by altering the neuro-endocrine regulation of food intake.

Adjunctive counseling for eating disorders

Further research is needed on the effects of eating disorders, including NES, on the outcome of bariatric surgery. Until such data are available, our research team recommends asking patients who have BED how concerned they are about their potential inability to control their binge eating after surgery [21]. We refer for cognitive behavioral treatment, before surgery, individuals who express significant anxiety or worry about binge eating; most do not. We instruct all patients to work closely with our program's dietitians before and after surgery and to contact them postoperatively whenever they feel they are eating too much or experiencing subjective loss of control of their food intake.

Quality of life

Extreme obesity almost universally results in decreased health-related quality of life (HRQL). This term refers to the burden of suffering and the limitations in physical, vocational, and social functioning associated with illness [62]. HRQL may be assessed by disease-specific measures, which seek to isolate the effects of a single illness (eg, diabetes-related quality of life), or by general measures, which do not reference a particular disease or condition. The Medical Outcomes Survey, Short Form 36 (SF-36) is the most commonly used instrument for assessing the impact of general health on daily functioning [63]. Frequently used obesity-specific instruments include the Impact of Weight on Quality of Life (IWQOL) scale and its short form, the IWQOL-Lite [64,65].

Regardless of the type of measure used, numerous studies have shown that excess weight is associated with significant impairments in HRQL and that the severity of impairment is related to the severity of obesity [13,66,67]. Thus, candidates for bariatric surgery report significantly worse HRQL than their less obese counterparts who seek behavioral and pharmacologic weight loss interventions [68]. Patients frequently report that the pervasiveness and severity of their impairments are their strongest motivators for seeking bariatric surgery. Additionally, impairments in HRQL may account for increased symptoms of depression among bariatric surgery candidates [13].

The large weight loss produced by bariatric surgery is associated with significant improvements in weight-related comorbidities, including type 2 diabetes, hypertension, and dyslipidemia [69]. As a result, patients undergoing bariatric surgery report significantly fewer impairments in HRQL postoperatively than similarly obese individuals who receive nonsurgical treatment [25,70]. We briefly review several areas of functioning that seem to be favorably affected by weight loss after bariatric surgery.

Physical function

The strain of carrying excess weight can impede even the most basic physical functions and personal care tasks [71,72]. Numerous investigations have found that extremely obese individuals report significant impairment in performing activities such as walking, climbing stairs, bathing, and dressing [71,72] and that such difficulties are among the most distressing aspects of their obesity [73]. The large weight losses achieved with bariatric surgery seem to normalize physical function and other aspects of quality of life. Nguyen and colleagues [74], for example, found that patients' physical function was significantly impaired before their undergoing open or laparoscopic gastric bypass. At 3- and 6-month postoperative assessments, physical function had improved to that of the general population. These patients had a mean preoperative BMI of approximately 48 kg/m^2 (range, 40–60 kg/m^2). O'Brien and colleagues [70] studied less obese patients (mean BMI, 33.7 kg/m^2; range, 30–35 kg/m^2) who underwent laparoscopic adjustable gastric banding. Patients' scores on all SF-36 scales fell in the significantly impaired range at baseline but rose to meet or exceed normative levels 2 years after surgery after a 22% reduction in initial weight. Physical functioning scores improved significantly more in surgically treated patients than in participants in this study who were randomly assigned to a program of very-low-calorie diet, pharmacotherapy, and behavior modification, which produced a 2-year loss of only 5.5% of initial weight [70].

A 1-year prospective study of patients undergoing bariatric surgery showed the extent to which mobility and functional capacity improved with weight loss [75]. Fifteen extremely obese women completed a 6-minute walk test before and 1 year after undergoing laparoscopic adjustable gastric banding. The investigators instructed participants to cover as much distance as possible during the assessments and measured heart rate, oxygen saturation, and perceived exertion before and after each test. As compared with their preoperative assessments, participants covered nearly one third more distance postoperatively and showed significant reductions in pre- and post-walk heart rate and perceived exertion. Increased capacity and ease of walking likely accounted for some of the improvements in physical function observed postoperatively.

Weight loss and improvements in physical function also may be associated with significant reductions in weight-related pain and correction (or improvement) of weight-related postural abnormalities that limit mobility. The SOS study found that "work-restricting" pain in the neck, back, hips, knees, and ankles and effort-related calf pain were significantly more common among obese persons than among the general population [76,77]. Patients who underwent bariatric surgery reported significantly greater improvement (or resolution) in these types of pain over 2 years than did similarly obese control subjects who received nonsurgical treatment. Surgically treated patients were significantly less likely to develop such pains. The reduction of pain in weight-bearing joints, such as the knees and ankles, seems to be more durable than the relief that patients initially report in their lower backs and non–weight-bearing body areas. Improvement in the former areas can be observed at least 6 years after bariatric surgery [76].

Occupational function

Persons who have significant limitations in their functional abilities and mobility could be expected to have impaired occupational function. Additionally, pervasive weight-related stigma may limit the occupational opportunities of extremely obese individuals [11]. Bariatric surgery candidates have reported significant preoperative and postoperative improvements in work-related activities. Two reviews found clear evidence of improvements in employment, as well as in job status, performance, and satisfaction after bariatric surgery [4,6].

The effect of bariatric surgery on missed work time is complex. Surgically treated participants in the SOS study had 35% more sick days in the year after treatment than patients in the control group [78]. The increased rate in patients undergoing bariatric surgery was likely attributable to recovery from the operation. In years 3 and 4, however, the surgically treated patients had significantly fewer days of sick leave, with the greatest effect observed among older (ie, 47–60 years of age) patients. Such data have not been reported for patients in the United States or Canada.

Body image and marital and sexual function

Body image dissatisfaction is common in overweight and obese individuals [3,5]. As early as 1967, Stunkard and Mendelson [79] described a group of obese patients with body image "disparagement" who believed their bodies were "ugly and despicable" and that others viewed them with hostility and contempt. Their body image disparagement took the form of an overwhelming preoccupation with their obesity, often to the exclusion of any other personal characteristics. More recently, Sarwer and colleagues [80] observed a similar phenomenon in 8% of obese individuals who enrolled in a clinical trial. This subset of individuals met criteria for body dysmorphic disorder, defined as a preoccupation with an imagined or slight defect in appearance that causes clinically significant distress or impairment in social, occupational, or other areas of functioning [81]. Patients who had this disorder scored an average of 13.2 on the Beck Depression Inventory (indicative of mild depression), compared with normal scores (ie, mean of 7.2) for patients who reported body image dissatisfaction but did not meet criteria for body dysmorphic disorder. Neither Stunkard's nor Sarwer's patients were candidates for bariatric surgery, and only a minority of surgery candidates present with body image disparagement of this degree.

Numerous studies have reported that weight loss after bariatric surgery is associated with marked improvements in body image [5,13,64–66,81]. An early study by Halmi and colleagues [82], found that 70% of patients reported severe body image disturbance before surgery, which fell to 4% after weight loss. Adami and colleagues [83] reported that 3 years after surgery, patients' scores on the Body Image Dissatisfaction subscale (of the Eating Disorders Inventory) and on the physical attractiveness and fear of fatness subscales (of the Body Attitudes Questionnaire) improved to the point that they did not differ significantly from values for normal weight-control subjects. Amelioration of body image is likely to be associated with improved social functioning as it was in the SOS study [25]. At a 2-year assessment, surgically treated patients reported that they were significantly less troubled than control participants by events such as going to restaurants or community activities, shopping for clothes, or being seen in a bathing suit. They also reported significantly greater satisfaction with personal relationships.

Marital and sexual function

Many patients present for bariatric surgery with the expectation that weight loss will improve their marital and sexual relationships, whereas others fear that changes in their weight and body shape may destabilize these relationships [3,5]. There have been few empirical studies of this issue, but most of the evidence suggests that improvements in relationship quality and satisfaction are more likely to improve than deteriorate [4–6]. Additionally, the effect of surgery seems to be a function of the quality of the existing relationship [84]. Postoperative marital problems are more likely attributable to a poor preoperative relationship than to the effects of the surgery. Nonproblematic relationships seem to remain stable or to improve.

Sexual function

Little is known about the effects of surgically induced weight loss on sexual function and satisfaction. Extremely obese persons report greater impairments in sexual quality of life than their less obese counterparts [85], and obese individuals—particularly women—seem to be stigmatized as potential sexual partners [86]. Additionally, researchers have shown obesity-related metabolic abnormalities were associated with sexual dysfunction and that erectile function improved in about one third of men who lost weight with lifestyle modification [87,88]. Given these findings, sexual quality of life in extremely obese men (and perhaps women) could be expected to improve after bariatric surgery. Controlled studies are needed to test this hypothesis.

Clinical concerns

The last section of this article addresses clinical problems for which there has been limited systematic research. These problems include (1) suboptimal weight loss, (2) vomiting and plugging, (3) gastric dumping, and (4) plastic surgery after weight loss. These problems are likely to attract more research attention with the continued growth of bariatric surgery.

Suboptimal weight loss

Patients typically lose 25% to 30% of initial body weight with GBP and 20% to 25% with restrictive procedures within the first 2 years postoperatively [69,89–93]. Approximately 20% of patients fail to obtain these losses [90,92,94]. Others begin to regain large amounts of weight within the first few postoperative years. These suboptimal results typically are attributed to poor adherence to the postoperative diet.

Several studies have suggested that patients struggle to adhere to the rigors of the postoperative diet [95–98]. Caloric intake often increases significantly over time [92,95,99–101]. For example, in the SOS trial [94], patients consumed approximately 2900 kcal/d before surgery. Their intake decreased to 1500 kcal/d 6 months after surgery but increased to approximately 2000 kcal/d 10 years later. This increase in caloric intake suggests the possible benefit of pre- or postoperative dietary counseling, particularly to improve adherence to the postoperative diet, thus maximizing weight loss. Such counseling makes intuitive sense, and investigations of its potential efficacy are in progress.

Vomiting and plugging

One third to two thirds of patients undergoing bariatric surgery report postoperative vomiting [46,52,102–107]. Vomiting is thought to occur most frequently during the first few postoperative months [108] but has been reported to occur for several years postoperatively [29,52,104,109,110]. This vomiting, whether reflexive or self-induced, does not seem to be a purging behavior (as seen in bulimia nervosa). Patients may vomit in response to intolerable foods or in an effort to clear food that has become lodged in the upper digestive track. This latter event, referred to as plugging, is typically the result of overeating, particularly of pasta, bread, and dry meats [46,52,103]. It has been reported in as many as 43% of patients for as long as 15 years postoperatively [52]. Although patients often attribute their vomiting to a physiologic problem, anecdotal reports suggest that vomiting is usually the result of consuming large portions or incomplete chewing of food. If physiologic causes for excessive vomiting have been ruled out, dietary counseling is recommended.

Gastric dumping

Gastric dumping, which encompasses a variety of symptoms including nausea, flushing, bloating, faintness, fatigue, and (often) severe diarrhea, may be the most undesirable postoperative event [52,92,93]. Patient reports suggest that it usually occurs after the consumption of foods high in sugar. These unpleasant symptoms should "encourage" patients, by means of aversive conditioning, to limit the intake of cakes, cookies, ice cream, and other sweets.

Despite its untoward symptoms, the occurrence of dumping has not been well documented. Studies suggest that it occurs in 50% to 70% of patients undergoing GBP [93,111]. Anecdotal reports suggest that it may not occur in all patients or may occur temporarily during the postoperative period [30].

Body contouring after bariatric surgery

According to the American Society of Plastic Surgeons, in 2005, approximately 68,000 patients underwent body contouring procedures after the massive weight loss typically associated with bariatric surgery [112]. The most common procedures were breast reduction procedures, which were performed on 31,277 patients. Extended abdominoplasty/lower body lift procedures, which are designed to eliminate the excessive skin around the abdomen and lower torso, were performed on 20,630 individuals. Upper arm lifts and thigh lifts were performed on 8,741 and 7,486 persons, respectively.

There is a rapidly growing body of knowledge related to the surgical aspects of these procedures [113]. Given the newness of this subspecialty within plastic surgery, we recommend that patients interested in body contouring seek treatment from board-certified plastic surgeons experienced with these challenging procedures. Little, however, is known about the psychological aspects of body contouring surgery [114]. Body image dissatisfaction is believed to play a central role in motivating people to undergo other plastic surgical procedures [115]. Patients undergoing bariatric surgery report improvements in body image after weight loss with behaviorally based programs and bariatric surgery [82,116–123]. Some patients undergoing bariatric surgery report residual body image dissatisfaction associated with loose, sagging skin of the breasts, abdomen, thighs, and arms after the massive weight loss [80,81]. This dissatisfaction likely motivates some individuals to seek plastic surgery to address these concerns.

Summary

Bariatric surgery is the most effective intervention for persons who have a BMI of 40 kg/m^2 or greater. It routinely induces weight losses of 25% to 30% of initial weight; such weight loss is associated with marked improvements in obesity-related comorbidities, including type 2 diabetes, hypertension, and sleep apnea. This article has shown that surgery-induced weight loss is generally associated with improvements in psychosocial status and HRQL, but changes in mental health after bariatric surgery are not as predictable as those in type 2 diabetes and related conditions. Weight loss should not be viewed as a treatment for major depression or the other significant psychiatric disorders that are observed in approximately 25% of persons who seek bariatric surgery. Researchers and clinicians are not able to predict which surgery patients will have suboptimal weight loss or suffer from clinically significant behavioral complications, including depression, binge eating, vomiting, or dumping. A minority of patients will report such problems postoperatively and will need the care of a multidisciplinary team that includes registered dietitians and mental health professionals who have expertise in weight management.

References

[1] Allison DB, Fontaine KR, Manson JE, et al. Annual deaths attributable to obesity in the United States. JAMA 1999;282:1530–8.

[2] Calle EE, Rodriguez C, Walker-Thurmond K, et al. Overweight, obesity, and mortality from cancer in a prospectively studied cohort of U.S. adults. N Engl J Med 2003;348: 1625–38.

[3] Wadden TA, Sarwer DB, Womble LG, et al. Psychosocial aspects of obesity and obesity surgery. Surg Clin North Am 2001;81:1001–24.

[4] Herpertz S, Kielmann R, Wolf AM, et al. Does obesity surgery improve psychosocial functioning? A systematic review. Int J Obes 2003;27:1300–14.

[5] Sarwer DB, Wadden TA, Fabricatore AF. Psychosocial and behavioral aspects of bariatric surgery. Obes Res 2005;13:639–48.

[6] Bocchieri LE, Meana M, Fisher BL. A review of psychosocial outcomes of surgery for morbid obesity. J Psychosom Res 2002;52(3):155–65.

[7] van Hout GC, Boekestein P, Fortuin FA, et al. Psychosocial functioning following bariatric surgery. Obes Surg 2006;16:787–94.

[8] Wadden TA, Butryn ML, Sarwer DB, et al. Comparison of psychosocial status in treatment-seeking women with class III vs. class I-II obesity. Obesity 2006;14(Suppl 2): 90S–8S.

[9] Swenson WM, Pearson JS, Osborne D. An MMPI source book: basic item, scale and pattern data on 50,000 medical patients. Minneapolis (MN): University of Minnesota Press; 1973.

[10] Onyike CU, Crum RM, Lee HB, et al. Is obesity associated with major depression? Results from the Third National Health and Nutrition Examination Survey. Am J Epidemiol 2003; 158:1139–47.

[11] Puhl R, Brownell KD. Bias, discrimination, and obesity. Obes Res 2001;9:788–805.

[12] Wadden TA, Stunkard AJ. Social and psychological consequences of obesity. Ann Intern Med 1985;103:1062–7.

[13] Fabricatore AN, Wadden TA, Sarwer DB, et al. Health-related quality of life and symptoms of depression in extremely obese persons seeking bariatric surgery. Obes Surg 2005; 15:304–9.

[14] Allison KC, Stunkard AJ. Obesity and eating disorders. Psychiatr Clin North Am 2005;28: 55–67.

[15] Yanovski SZ, Nelson JE, Dubbert BK, et al. Association of binge eating disorder and psychiatric comorbidity in obese subjects. Am J Psychiatry 1993;150:1472–9.

[16] Herpertz S, Kielmann R, Wolf AM, et al. Do psychosocial variables predict weight loss or mental health after obesity surgery? A systematic review. Obes Res 2004;12:1554–69.

[17] van Hout GC, Verschure SK, van Heck GL. Psychosocial predictors of success following bariatric surgery. Obes Surg 2005;15:552–60.

[18] Clark MM, Balsiger BM, Sletten CD, et al. Psychosocial factors and 2-year outcome following bariatric surgery for weight loss. Obes Surg 2003;13:739–45.

[19] Averbukh Y, Heshka S, El-Shoreya H, et al. Depression score predicts weight loss following Roux-en-Y gastric bypass. Obes Surg 2003;13:833–6.

[20] Buchwald H, Consensus Conference Panel. Bariatric surgery for morbid obesity: health implications for patients, health professionals, and third-party payers. J Am Coll Surg 2005; 200:593–604.

[21] Wadden TA, Sarwer DB. Behavioral assessment of candidates for bariatric surgery: a patient-oriented approach. Obesity 2006;14(Suppl 2):53S–62S.

[22] Wadden TA, Foster GD. Weight and lifestyle inventory (WALI). Obesity 2006;14(Suppl 2): 99S–118S.

[23] Beck AT, Steer RA, Brown GK. Beck depression inventory II (BDI-II) manual. San Antonio (TX): Harcourt Brace & Company; 1993.

[24] Fabricatore AN, Crerand CE, Wadden TA, et al. How do mental health professionals evaluate candidates for bariatric surgery? Survey results. Obes Surg 2006;16:567–73.

[25] Karlsson J, Sjostrom L, Sullivan M. Swedish obese subjects (SOS): an intervention study of obesity: two-year follow-up of health-related quality of life (HRQL) and eating behavior after gastric surgery for severe obesity. Int J Obes 1998;22:113–26.

[26] Sullivan M, Karlsson J, Sjostrom L, et al. Why quality of life measures should be used in the treatment of patients with obesity. In: Bjorntrop P, editor. International textbook of obesity. London: John Wiley and Sons; 2001. p. 485–510.

[27] Dixon JB, Dixon ME, O'Brien PE. Depression in association with severe obesity: changes with weight loss. Arch Intern Med 2003;163:2058–65.

[28] Waters GS, Pories WJ, Swanson MS, et al. Long-term studies of mental health after the Greenville gastric bypass operation for morbid obesity. Am J Surg 1991;161:154–8.

[29] Powers PS, Rosemurgy A, Boyd F, et al. Outcome of gastric restriction procedures: weight, psychiatric diagnoses, and satisfaction. Obes Surg 1997;7:471–7.

[30] Hsu LK, Benotti PN, Dwyer J, et al. Nonsurgical factors that influence the outcome of bariatric surgery: a review. Psychosom Med 1998;60:338–46.

[31] Higa KD, Boone KB, Ho T. Complications of the laparoscopic Roux-en-Y gastric bypass: 1,040 patients—what have we learned? Obes Surg 2000;10:509–13.

[32] Dong C, Li W-D, Li D, et al. Extreme obesity is associated with attempted suicides: results from a family study. Int J Obes 2006;30:388–90.

[33] Carpenter KM, Hasin DS, Allison DB, et al. Relationships between obesity and DSM-IV major depressive disorder, suicide ideation, and suicide attempts: results from a general population study. Am J Public Health 2000;90:251–7.

[34] Omalu BI, Cho P, Shakir AM, et al. Suicides following bariatric surgery for the treatment of obesity. Surg Obes Relat Dis 2005;1:447–9.

[35] Spitzer RL, Yanovski S, Wadden T, et al. Binge eating disorder: its further validation in a multi-site study. Int J Eat Disord 1993;13:137–53.

[36] Kalarchian MA, Wilson GT, Brolin RE, et al. Binge eating in bariatric surgery patients. Int J Eat Disord 1998;23:89–92.

[37] Hsu LKG, Mulliken B, McDonagh B, et al. Binge eating disorder in extreme obesity. Int J Obes 2002;26:1398–403.

[38] de Zwaan M, Mitchell JE, Howell LM, et al. Characteristics of morbidly obese patients before gastric bypass surgery. Compr Psychiatry 2003;44:428–34.

[39] Spitzer RL, Devlin M, Walsh TB, et al. Binge eating disorder: a multi-site field trial of the diagnostic criteria. Int J Eat Disord 1992;11:191–203.

[40] Mussell MP, Peterson CB, Weller CL, et al. Differences in body image and depression among obese women with and without binge eating disorder. Obes Res 1996;4:431–9.

[41] Specker S, de Zwaan M, Raymond N, et al. Psychopathology in subgroups of obese women with and without binge eating disorder. Compr Psychiatry 1994;35:185–90.

[42] Telch C, Stice E. Psychiatric comorbidity in non-clinical sample of women with binge eating disorder. J Consult Clin Psychol 1998;66:768–76.

[43] Wilfley DE, Welch RR, Stein RI, et al. A randomized comparison of group cognitive behavior therapy and group interpersonal psychotherapy for the treatment of overweight individuals with binge eating disorder. Arch Gen Psychiatry 2002;59:713–21.

[44] Allison KC, Wadden TA, Sarwer DB, et al. Night eating syndrome and binge eating disorder among persons seeking bariatric surgery: prevalence and related features. Obesity 2006; 14(Suppl 2):77S–82S.

[45] Adami GF, Meneghelli A, Scopinaro N. Night eating and binge eating disorder in obese patients. Int J Eat Disord 1999;25:335–8.

[46] Powers PS, Perez A, Boyd F, et al. Eating pathology before and after bariatric surgery: a prospective study. Int J Eat Disord 1999;25:293–300.

[47] Stunkard AJ, Allison KC. Two forms of disordered eating in obesity: binge eating and night eating. Int J Obes Relat Metab Disord 2003;27:1–12.

[48] Dymek MP, le Grange D, Neven K, et al. Quality of life and psychosocial adjustment in patients after Roux-en-Y gastric bypass: a brief report. Obes Surg 2001;11:32–9.

[49] Hsu LKG, Betancourt S, Sullivan SP. Eating disturbances before and after vertical banded gastroplasty: a pilot study. Int J Eat Dis 1996;19:23–34.

[50] Hsu LKG, Betancourt S, Sullivan SP. Eating disturbances and outcome of gastric bypass surgery: a pilot study. Int J Eat Dis 1997;21:385–90.

[51] Kalarchian MA, Wilson GT, Brolin RE, et al. Effects of bariatric surgery on binge eating and related psychopathology. Eat Weight Disord 1999;4:1–5.

[52] Mitchell JE, Lancaster KL, Burgard MA, et al. Long-term follow-up of patients' status after gastric bypass. Obes Surg 2001;11:464–8.

[53] Busetto L, Valente P, Pisent C, et al. Eating pattern in the first year following adjustable silicone gastric banding (ASGB) for morbid obesity. Int J Obes Relat Metab Disord 1996;20:539–46.

[54] Busetto L, Segato G, De Marchi F, et al. Outcome predictors in morbidly obese recipients of an adjustable gastric band. Obes Surg 2002;12:83–92.

[55] Malone M, Alger-Mayer S. Binge status and quality of life after gastric bypass surgery: a one-year study. Obes Res 2004;12:473–81.

[56] Devlin MJ, Goldfein JA, Flancbaum L, et al. Surgical management of obese patients with eating disorders: a survey of current practice. Obes Surg 2004;14:1252–7.

[57] Kalarchian MA, Marcus MD, Wilson GT, et al. Binge eating among gastric bypass patients at long-term follow-up. Obes Surg 2002;12:270–5.

[58] Lang T, Hauser R, Buddeberg C, et al. Impact of gastric banding on eating behavior and weight. Obes Surg 2002;12:100–7.

[59] Cummings DE, Weigle DS, Frayo RS, et al. Plasma ghrelin levels after diet-induced weight loss or gastric bypass surgery. N Engl J Med 2002;346:1623–30.

[60] Morton GJ, Cummings DE, Baskin DG, et al. Central nervous system control of food intake and body weight. Nature 2006;443:289–95.

[61] Cummings DE. Ghrelin and the short- and long-term regulation of appetite and body weight. Physiol Behav 2006;89:71–84.

[62] Wadden TA, Phelan S. Assessment of quality of life in obese individuals. Obes Res 2002; 10S:50S–7S.

[63] Ware JE, Snow KK, Kosinski M, et al. SF-36 Health Survey: manual and interpretation guide. Boston: The Health Institute, New England Medical Center; 1993.

[64] Kolotkin RL, Head S, Hamilton M, et al. Assessing impact of weight on quality of life. Obes Res 1995;3:49–56.

[65] Kolotkin RL, Crosby RD, Kosloski KD, et al. Development of a brief measure to assess quality of life in obesity. Obes Res 2001;9:102–11.

[66] Kolotkin RL, Meter K, Williams GR. Quality of life and obesity. Obes Rev 2001;2:219–29.

[67] Fontaine KR, Barofsky I. Obesity and health-related quality of life. Obes Rev 2001;2: 173–82.

[68] Kolotkin RL, Crosby RD, Williams GR. Health-related quality of life varies among obese subgroups. Obes Res 2002;10:748–56.

[69] Maggard MA, Shugarman LR, Suttorp M, et al. Meta-analysis: surgical treatment of obesity. Ann Intern Med 2005;142:547–59.

[70] O'Brien PE, Dixon JB, Laurie C, et al. Treatment of mild to moderate obesity with laparoscopic adjustable gastric banding or an intensive medical program. Ann Intern Med 2006; 144:625–33.

[71] Larsson UE, Mattsson E. Perceived disability and observed functional limitations in obese women. Int J Obes Relat Metab Disord 2001;25:1705–12.

[72] Larsson UE, Mattsson E. Functional limitations linked to high body mass index, age and current pain in obese women. Int J Obes Relat Metab Disord 2001;25:893–9.

[73] Duval K, Marceau P, Lescelleur O, et al. Health-related quality of life in morbid obesity. Obes Surg 2006;16:574–9.

[74] Nguyen NT, Goldman C, Rosenquist J, et al. Laparoscopic versus open gastric bypass: a randomized study of outcomes, quality of life, and costs. Ann Surg 2001;234:279–89.

[75] Maniscalco M, Zedda A, Giardiello C, et al. Effect of bariatric surgery on the six-minute walk test in severe uncomplicated obesity. Obes Surg 2006;16:836–41.

[76] Peltonen M, Lindroos AK, Torgerson JS. Musculoskeletal pain in the obese: a comparison with a general population and long-term changes after conventional and surgical obesity treatment. Pain 2003;104:549–57.

[77] Karason K, Peltonen M, Lindroos AK, et al. Effort-related calf pain in the obese and long-term changes after surgical obesity treatment. Obes Res 2005;13:137–45.

[78] Narbro K, Argen G, Jonsson E, et al. Sick leave and disability pension before and after treatment for obesity: a report from the Swedish Obese Subjects (SOS) study. Int J Obes Relat Metab Disord 1999;23:619–24.

[79] Stunkard A, Mendelson M. Obesity and the body image: characteristics of disturbances in the body image of some obese persons. Am J Psychiatry 1967;123:1296–300.

[80] Sarwer DB, Wadden TA, Foster GD. Assessment of body image dissatisfaction in obese women: specificity, severity, and clinical significance. J Consult Clin Psychol 1998;66: 651–4.

[81] Sarwer DB, Thompson JK, Cash TF. Body image and obesity in adulthood. Psychiatr Clin North Am 2005;28:69–87.

[82] Halmi KA, Long M, Stunkard AJ, et al. Psychiatric diagnosis of morbidly obese gastric bypass patients. Am J Psychiatry 1980;134:470–2.

[83] Adami GF, Gandolfo P, Campostano A, et al. Body image and body weight in obese patients. Int J Eat Disord 1998;24:299–306.

[84] Rand CS, Kuldau JM, Robbins L. Surgery for obesity and marriage quality. JAMA 1982; 247:1419–22.

[85] Kolotkin RL, Binks M, Crosby RD, et al. Obesity and sexual quality of life. Obesity 2006; 14:472–9.

[86] Chen EY, Brown M. Obesity stigma in sexual relationships. Obes Res 2005;13:1393–7.

[87] Esposito K, Giugliano D. Obesity, the metabolic syndrome, and sexual dysfunction. Int J Impot Res 2005;17:391–8.

[88] Esposito K, Giugliano F, Di Palo C, et al. Effect of lifestyle changes on erectile dysfunction in obese men: a randomized controlled trial. JAMA 2004;291:2978–84.

[89] Benotti PN, Forse RA. The role of gastric surgery in the multidisciplinary management of severe obesity. Am J Surg 1995;169:361–7.

[90] Brolin RE, Kenler HA, Gorman RC, et al. The dilemma of outcome assessment after operations for morbid obesity. Surgery 1989;105:337–46.

[91] MacLean LD, Rhode BM, Sampalis J, et al. Results of the surgical treatment of obesity. Am J Surg 1993;165:155–9.

[92] Sugerman HJ, Londrey GL, Kellum JM. Weight loss with vertical banded gastroplasty and Roux-Y gastric bypass for morbid obesity with selective vs. random assignment. Am J Surg 1989;157:93–102.

[93] Sugerman HJ, Starkey JV, Birkenhauer R. A randomized prospective trial of gastric bypass versus vertical banded gastroplasty for morbid obesity and their effects on sweets versus non-sweets eaters. Ann Surg 1987;205:613–24.

[94] Sjostrom L, Lindroos AK, Peltonen M, et al. Swedish Obese Subjects Study Scientific Group. Lifestyle, diabetes and cardiovascular risk factors 10 years after bariatric surgery. N Engl J Med 2004;351:2683–93.

[95] Anderson T, Larsen U. Dietary outcomes in obese patients treated with a gastroplasty program. Am J Clin Nutr 1989;50:1328–40.

[96] MacLean LD, Rhode BM, Shizgal HM. Nutrition following gastric operations for morbid obesity. Ann Surg 1983;198:347–55.

[97] Miskowiak J, Honore K, Larsen L, et al. Food intake before and after gastroplasty for morbid obesity. Scand J Gastroenterol 1985;20:925–8.

[98] Naslund I, Jarnmark I, Anderson H. Dietary intake before and after gastric bypass and gastroplasty for morbid obesity in women. Int J Obes Relat Metab Disord 1988;12: 503–13.

[99] Kenler HA, Brolin RE, Cody RC. Changes in eating behavior after horizontal gastroplasty and Roux-en-Y gastric bypass. Am J Clin Nutr 1990;52:87–92.

[100] Lindroos AK, Lissner L, Sjostrom L. Weight change in relation to intake of sugar and sweet foods before and after weight reducing gastric surgery. Int J Obes Relat Metab Disord 1996; 20:634–43.

[101] Moize V, Geliebter A, Gluck ME, et al. Obese patients have inadequate protein intake related to protein intolerance up to 1 year following Roux-en-Y gastric bypass. Obes Surg 2003;13:23–8.

[102] Brolin RE, Robertson LB, Kenler HA, et al. Weight loss and dietary intake after vertical banded gastroplasty and Roux-en-Y gastric bypass. Ann Surg 1994;220:782–90.

[103] Kinzl JF, Trefalt E, Fiala M, et al. Psychotherapeutic treatment of morbidly obese patients after gastric banding. Obes Surg 2002;12:292–4.

[104] Wyss C, Laurent-Jaccard A, Burckhardt P, et al. Long-term results on quality of life of surgical treatment of obesity with vertical banded gastroplasty. Obes Surg 1995;5: 387–92.

[105] Halverson JD, Zuckerman GR, Koehler RE, et al. Gastric bypass for morbid obesity: a medical-surgical assessment. Ann Surg 1981;194:152–60.

[106] Pekkarinen T, Koskela K, Huikuri K, et al. Long-term results of gastroplasty for morbid obesity: binge-eating as a predictor of poor outcome. Obes Surg 1994;4:248–55.

[107] Pessina A, Andreoli M, Vassallo C. Adaptability and compliance of the obese patient to restrictive gastric surgery in the short term. Obes Surg 2001;11:459–63.

[108] Stunkard AJ, Foster GD, Glassman J, et al. Retro-spective exaggeration of symptoms: vomiting after gastric surgery for obesity. Psychosom Med 1985;47:150–5.

[109] Adami GF, Gandolfo P, Bauer B, et al. Binge eating in massively obese patients undergoing bariatric surgery. Int J Eat Disord 1995;17:45–50.

[110] Balsiger BM, Poggio JL, Mai J, et al. Ten and more years after vertical banded gastroplasty as primary operation for morbid obesity. J Gastrointest Surg 2000;4:598–605.

[111] Pories WJ, Swanson MS, MacDonald KG, et al. Who would have thought it? An operation proves to be the most effective therapy for adult-onset diabetes mellitus. Ann Surg 1995; 222:339–52.

[112] American Society of Plastic Surgeons. 2005 National plastic surgery statistics. Arlington Heights (IL): ASPS; 2006.

[113] Rohrich RJ, Kenkel JM. Body contouring after massive weight loss supplement. Plast Reconstr Surg 2006;117:S1–86.

[114] Sarwer DB, Thompson JK, Mitchell JE, et al. Psychological considerations of the bariatric surgery patient undergoing body contouring surgery. Plast Reconstr Surg, in press.

[115] Sarwer DB, Pruzinsky T, Cash TF, et al. Psychological aspects of reconstructive and cosmetic plastic surgery: empirical, clinical, and ethical issues. Philadelphia: Lippincott, Williams, and Wilkins; 2006.

[116] Dixon JB, Dixon ME, O'Brien PE. Body image: appearance orientation and evaluation in the severely obese. Obes Surg 2002;12:65–71.

[117] Gentry K, Halverson JD, Heisler S. Psychologic assessment of morbidly obese patients undergoing gastric bypass: a comparison of preoperative and postoperative adjustment. Surgery 1984;95:215–20.

[118] Solow C, Silberfarb PM, Swift K. Psychosocial effects of intestinal bypass surgery for severe obesity. N Engl J Med 1974;290:300–4.

[119] Foster GD, Wadden TA, Vogt RA. Body image in obese women before, during, and after weight loss treatment. Health Psychol 1997;16:226–9.

[120] Cash TF. Body-image attitudes among obese enrollees in a commercial weight-loss program. Percept Mot Skills 1993;77:1099–103.

[121] Wadden TA, Foster GD, Sarwer DB, et al. Dieting and the development of eating disorders in obese women: results of a randomized controlled trial. Am J Clin Nutr 2004;80:560–8.

[122] Camps MA, Zervos E, Goode S, et al. Impact of bariatric surgery on body image perception and sexuality in morbidly obese patients and their partners. Obes Surg 1996;6:356–60.

[123] Neven K, Dymek M, leGrange D, et al. The effects of Roux-en-Y gastric bypass surgery on body image. Obes Surg 2002;12:265–9.

THE MEDICAL
CLINICS
OF NORTH AMERICA

Med Clin N Am 91 (2007) 471–483

Outpatient Complications Encountered Following Roux-en-Y Gastric Bypass

Peter P. Lopez, MD[a], Nilesh A. Patel, MD[a],*,
Lisa S. Koche, MD[b,c]

[a]Department of Surgery, University of Texas Health Science Center San Antonio, 7703 Floyd
Curl Drive, MC7740, San Antonio, TX 78229, USA
[b]Spectra Complete Healthcare, University of South Florida, 509 South Armenia Avenue,
Suite #302, Tampa, FL 33609, USA
[c]Weight Management and Metabolic Health Center, P.O. Box 1289,
Suite F-145, Tampa, FL 33601, USA

Over the next 10 years, an exponential growth in weight loss surgery has been predicted. By the year 2010, over 250,000 procedures per year are projected to be performed in the United States alone. This rapid growth rate coincides with a focus by payers and surgical societies to centralize care with "centers of excellence" designations. The concept of centralization of care is based on reports in which the perioperative and long-term outcomes of procedures are better at high-volume centers and when performed by high-volume surgeons. The best example of how this model has been implemented is the 2006 National Care Determination in which access to care for Medicare recipients was limited to centers of excellence as designated by the Surgical Review Corporation and the American Society of Bariatric Surgery or the American College of Surgeons.

With outcomes being the major focus, the ramifications of such designations in the short term equate to limited access to care. Currently, 13 states have no such designated centers. Many of the states with designated centers have two or fewer centers to serve the entire state. These limitations immediately impact the referring physician, placing a greater onus on these physicians in the outpatient management of the post gastric bypass patient. This article outlines the incidence, clinical presentation, and management of commonly encountered complications following gastric bypass.

* Corresponding author. P.O. Box 691996, San Antonio, TX 78229.
E-mail address: drpatel@bypassdoc.com (N.A. Patel).

0025-7125/07/$ - see front matter © 2007 Elsevier Inc. All rights reserved.
doi:10.1016/j.mcna.2007.01.008 *medical.theclinics.com*

Overview of the management of complications

The key to the management of complications is prevention. As mentioned in a separate article in this issue by Kuruba and colleagues, a multidisciplinary approach to the patient is needed in the preoperative assessment. The focus of this multidisciplinary team should be appropriate patient selection, the identification and optimization of comorbidities, and patient education. When complications arise after bariatric surgery, a low threshold of suspicion is required to make an early diagnosis. Management of acute complications in morbidly obese patients remains a challenge because they often do not manifest many clinical signs and symptoms when they become ill. Also, morbidly obese patients have limited physiologic reserve and often do not manifest fevers, abdominal pain, or an increased white blood cell count. Physicians caring for postoperative bariatric patients must maintain a high index of suspicion to prevent, recognize, diagnose, and treat postoperative complications.

Abdominal pain following gastric bypass

Abdominal pain following gastric bypass has an extensive list of differential diagnoses. Although commonly occurring disease states such as gastroenteritis cannot be excluded, one must first consider conditions specific to, or as a consequence of, gastric bypass. Table 1 lists common causes of abdominal pain following gastric bypass. As seen in Table 2, as is true in nonoperative patients, abdominal pain can be differentiated by the location and character of the pain as well as the timing of the symptoms relative to meals and the initial surgery. Each condition is discussed individually in the following sections.

Biliary disease

Risk factors for gallstone formation include obesity and rapid weight loss. Bile stasis can lead to sludge and gallstone formation. Shiffman and colleagues [1] reported a 50% rate of gallbladder sludge formation 6 months after gastric bypass. The incidence of symptomatic gallbladder disease after bariatric surgery ranges from 3% to 30% [2]. Management of gallbladder disease in obese patients remains debatable. Some clinicians routinely screen obese patients for gallstones and remove their gallbladders at the time of

Table 1
Incidence of common causes of abdominal pain following gastric bypass

Cause of abdominal pain	Incidence (%)
Biliary disease	3–30
Gastrojejunal stricture	0.6–27
Marginal ulceration	1–16
Internal hernia	2–5
Constipation (dehydration)	5–25

Table 2
Differentiating common causes of abdominal pain following gastric bypass

Cause of abdominal pain	Location	Time from surgery	Time from meal
Biliary disease	Epigastric/right upper quadrant	>6 mo	Hours
Gastrojejunal stricture	Epigastric	<3 mo	<10 min
Marginal ulceration	Mid-epigastric, radiates to back	<3 mo	No relation
Internal hernia	Left upper quadrant	>1 y	>10 min
Constipation	Left lower quadrant	Any time	No relation

bypass if stones are found or patients have had prior gallbladder symptoms. Others routinely recommend the removal of the gallbladder at the time of bariatric surgery [3], which can increase the length of the procedure up to 50 minutes [4]. Although others will wait until symptomatic gallbladder disease develops in the patient and then remove the gallbladder, Sugarman and colleagues [5] showed that the use of 600 mg of ursodiol daily for 6 months decreased the rate of gallstone formation after gastric bypass from 32%, with no treatment to 2%.

The presentation of symptomatic cholithiasis following gastric bypass is no different than in the nonoperative patient. Postprandial right upper quadrant pain radiating to the back and right shoulder is the hallmark. The diagnosis can be confounded by marginal ulceration or gastrojejunostomy stricture if epigastric pain is the only presenting symptom. In this case, the timing of the symptoms relative to eating and the surgery are important. Biliary disease is most often present greater than 6 months from the time of surgery, and the pain is usually a few hours after eating as opposed to immediately after. Ulcerations and strictures usually present less than 3 months postoperatively and are associated with dysphagia to solids, and the onset of pain is usually just a few minutes after eating.

The diagnosis of symptomatic biliary disease remains the same. A right upper quadrant ultrasound is the best initial test. In addition, a white blood cell count and liver function panel are also mandatory because the management of post gastric bypass choledocholithiasis is a more difficult problem because these patients can no longer have an endoscopic retrograde cholangiopancreatography (ERCP) performed. If the patient has had a gastrostomy performed in the past, an ERCP can be performed through a dilated gastrostomy site. A laparoscopic transgastric approach for ERCP has also been described [6]. Occasionally, an open common bile duct exploration may need to be performed.

Gastrojejunal stricture

Patients presenting within 3 to 10 weeks after surgery with nausea and vomiting commonly have obstruction from a stricture occurring at their gastrojejunostomy. These lesions result from ischemia at the site of the anastomosis or from small subclinical anastomotic leaks. In one study in patients who had their gastrojejunostomy performed with a circular stapler, the use of a larger 25-mm anvil resulted in less strictures when compared with the use of a smaller 21-mm anvil [7]. A Gastrografin upper gastrointestinal series can make the diagnosis.

Patients present with dysphagia to solids greater than liquids. Epigastric discomfort is noted usually after less than 10 minutes of eating. Patients are treated by endoscopic dilatation of their stricture. Marginal ulcerations can present in a similar manner, but the degree of dysphagia is usually worse with a stricture, and pain is often seen with solids and liquids in the case of ulceration. In the authors' practice, dilations are performed serially until dysphagia to solids resolves. Serial dilation reduces the chances of perforation. Maximal dilation in the authors' practice is to 15 mm to reduce the chances of perforation and not to diminish the degree of restriction at the level of the gastrojejunostomy. Strictures following ulcerations should be dilated more cautiously because there is a higher risk of perforation in these patients.

Marginal ulceration

Marginal ulcers occur at the gastrojejunal anastomosis. The incidence ranges between 1% and 16% after gastric bypass [8]. Nausea, vomiting, epigastric pain, dysphagia to solids, and occult gastrointestinal bleeding are common presenting symptoms of marginal ulcers. Occasionally, marginal ulcers are the first sign of a gastrogastric fistula. This presentation is very similar to gastrojejunostomy strictures and is best differentiated by endoscopy.

The causes of marginal ulceration are tension, ischemia, staple line breakdown, peptic ulcer disease, outlet obstruction, stasis, and irritating medications. Non-steriodal anti-inflammatory medications (NSAIDs) and *Helicobacter pylori* have been associated with the development of marginal ulcers. Patients who were screened and treated preoperatively for *H pylori* had a significantly lower incidence of marginal ulcers at 3 years (2.4%) when compared with those who were not screened or treated [9]. Alcohol and smoking have also been associated with marginal ulcer formation [10]. The diagnosis is made when performing an upper endoscopy on patients with symptoms consistent for ulcers. These ulcers can usually be treated conservatively with protein pump inhibitors, H_2 blockade, or sucralfate therapy [11]. Treatment should be for at least 6 to 8 weeks with endoscopic confirmation of healing. Cessation of NSAIDs and smoking also help heal these ulcers. If marginal ulcers remain untreated, they can lead to stricture formation of the gastroenterostomy and gastric outlet obstruction [12]. For intractable marginal ulcers caused from tension on the anastomosis or ulcers associated with foreign bodies (including sutures) that do not heal and continue to cause pain, a reoperation with resection of the ulcer and revision of the gastroenterostomy may be indicated.

Intestinal obstruction and internal hernias

Intestinal obstruction after bariatric surgery can be caused by adhesions, internal hernias, anastomotic strictures, intussusception, and volvulus or kinking of the small bowel. The most common cause of small bowel obstruction after open bariatric procedures is adhesions. The incidence of bowel obstruction after open gastric bypass has been reported to be 1% to 3% [13].

Internal hernias remain the most common cause of small bowel obstruction after laparoscopic gastric bypass surgery. Comeau and colleagues [14] reported an incidence of internal hernias after laparoscopic bariatric surgery of 3.3%. Internal hernias commonly arise from three sites: (1) the space at the mesenteric defect of the distal small bowel anastomosis; (2) Peterson's space, the space behind the Roux limb; and (3) the space between the transverse mesocolic window. Antecolic placement of the Roux limb is associated with a lower risk (0.43%) of internal hernias when compared with retrocolic placement (4.5%) [15]. The most common site for internal hernias after a retrocolic gastric bypass is the mesocolic tunnel; after an antecolic gastric bypass, it is in Peterson's space. These internal hernias can result in a closed bowel obstruction, which if not diagnosed and treated promptly can lead to a fatal outcome. Internal hernias arise after laparoscopic procedures because few adhesions are formed when compared with open procedures and because many surgeons fail to close these defects using continuous nonabsorbable suture. Furthermore, rapid weight loss results in elongation of the mesentery and laxity of the mesenteric defect, facilitating hernia formation. Common presenting symptoms of internal herniation are intermittent epigastric pain, sometimes radiating to the back and occasionally postprandial. The pain can vary in intensity from mild to severe. Diagnosis of an internal hernia can be made by a preoperative CT scan or upper gastrointestinal contrast study; however, Higa and colleagues [16] showed that 20% of internal hernias are not always demonstrated by radiographic studies preoperatively. If the symptoms persist after a negative radiologic work-up, strong consideration needs to be given to performing a diagnostic laparoscopic exploration to rule out an internal hernia. Reduction of the herniated bowel and suture closure of the hernia space is usually all that is need for correction. If the herniated bowel has been compromised, necrotic bowel will need to be resected.

Intestinal obstructions may be partial or complete. Patients present with mild to severe, intermittent, or constant epigastric abdominal pain. Patients will occasionally have nausea and vomiting as well as obstipation. The clinician must diagnose a small bowel obstruction to prevent complications. Any patient who presents with nonspecific crampy abdominal pain after gastric bypass should be suspected to have a bowel obstruction. In the case of an internal hernia, patients will often recall similar episodes in the past that were self-limited. In addition, they will report that the symptoms are aggravated after eating. The cramping is usually worse in the left upper quadrant and is worst 10 to 30 minutes after eating.

If the patient has severe abdominal pain, he or she may have ischemic bowel. These patients differ from other postoperative surgical patients in whom the cause of obstruction is adhesions, which may justify an initial non-operative approach to the obstruction. All postoperative bariatric patients who present with an intestinal obstruction need to be evaluated quickly. If the precise cause of the obstruction cannot be determined, the patient should undergo an open or laparoscopic exploration to identify the cause of the pain and obstruction. This early and aggressive approach to obstruction after gastric bypass will prevent bowel necrosis and perforation [16].

Early obstruction of the biliopancreatic limb secondary to narrowing of the suture line or kinking of the bowel at the jejunojejunostomy can result in acute dilatation of the gastric remnant. This complication is rare (0.6%) [17] but can be catastrophic. This closed loop obstruction can lead to gastric perforation and hemodynamic instability. Patients present with severe unrelenting epigastric pain, hiccups, and gastric dilatation. This type of obstruction is seen most often in the perioperative period. Late obstructions of this limb can be diagnosed by a CT scan revealing a dilated gastric remnant and duodenum. Laboratory values may demonstrate a presentation consistent with obstructive jaundice. Treatment includes urgent percutaneous gastrostomy tube decompression followed by reduction of the underlying biliary limb obstruction.

Postoperative nausea and vomiting

Nausea and vomiting are signs and symptoms that arise from many different causes and can occur any time after bariatric surgery. This symptom complex remains the most common complaint following the initiation of a soft diet. Box 1 summarizes the most common causes of nausea and vomiting following gastric bypass. Vomiting occurs most commonly during the first few months after surgery. It often results from overeating or not chewing food properly. Patients can have nausea and vomiting from medications such as NSAIDs, antidepressants, potassium replacement, and narcotics. Pills can get stuck in the esophagus or at the gastric outlet. Motion sickness and pregnancy can also lead to nausea and vomiting. Unpleasant smells or food tastes can lead to nausea and vomiting. Common gastrointestinal causes of nausea and vomiting leading to a blocked or markedly stenosed gastric pouch are marginal ulceration, pouch gastritis, gastric ischemia, band slippage, and a foreign body bezoar. An upper gastrointestinal study along with the performance of an esophagogastroduodenoscopy will make the diagnosis of these causes of nausea and vomiting. Strictures of the gastroenterostomy can be dilated with relief of symptoms.

Box 1. Common causes of nausea and vomiting after gastric bypass

Overeating and poor eating habits
Gastrojejunostomy stricture
Gastric remnant dysmotility
Biliary dyskinesia
Medication related
Candidal esophagitis
Dehydration due to secondary illness
Marginal ulceration
Middle ear disturbance
Vitamin B_1 deficiency

Another important cause of persistent nausea and vomiting along with Wernicke-Korsakoff encephalopathy or profound irreversible peripheral neuropathy is the development of vitamin B_1 deficiency. This form of severe vomiting can easily be corrected with replacement of vitamin B_1. Zinc deficiency can cause nausea along with dysosmia and dysgeusia.

Because the list of differentials is extensive, the work-up can be tedious. In the authors' practice, the initial work-up includes a detailed diet history. If the patient is not able to tolerate solid food at all but can tolerate liquids, the mechanics of eating are reviewed with them. We emphasize eating no more than six to eight bites of food per meal, chewing each bite at least 3 minutes, and not drinking 30 minutes before and after meals. In addition, we confirm that the patient is continuing their proton pump inhibitor, which is used empirically for 3 months. The patient is instructed to take a preparation such as bismuth subsalicylate (Pepto-Bismol) or calcium carbonate with magnesium hydroxide (Mylanta) three times a day before meals. This regimen addresses eating mechanics and empirically treats an ulcer.

If the patient cannot tolerate liquids or if the previously described regimen fails after 3 to 4 days of treatment, an endoscopy is indicated. If a stricture or ulcer is diagnosed, *H pylori* titers are checked. If the endoscopy is negative and nausea and vomiting are persistent, a trial of metoclopromide hydrochloride (Reglan) is initiated. A trial of Reglan can also be considered empirically if the patient has persistent nausea even when they are taking nothing by mouth.

With persistence of symptoms at this point, rare causes of nausea and vomiting should be considered. The authors' initial test would be a gallbladder ultrasound followed by a study with cholecystokinin and lidofenin (CCK-HIDA) if the ultrasound is normal. As mentioned earlier, in the authors' series, biliary dyskinesia was a common cause of persistent nausea and vomiting. If the biliary work-up is negative, the patient is referred to an ear, nose, and throat specialist. One may also consider an empiric trial of fluconazole (Diflucan), 200 mg per day. Anecdotal reports of candidal esophagitis as a cause of persistent nausea and vomiting have been discussed at surgical meetings.

During the work-up process, which can be lengthy, appropriate nutritional support should be provided. At the time of endoscopy, the authors empirically give each patient a multivitamin intravenously and 1 mg of vitamin B_1. As outpatients, patients are started on protein shakes and a pureed diet. Rarely, hyperalimentation is needed, but a low threshold should be maintained for chronic cases. The authors have noted patients with severe dehydration from gastroenteritis and other causes presenting with nausea and vomiting despite the instigating cause having resolved. In such cases, simple intravenous hydration resolved the nausea and vomiting.

Thromboembolism

Pulmonary embolus occurs in approximately 1.4% to 2.6% of all postoperative bariatric surgery patients [18]. It remains a common cause of death in these patients, with an overall mortality rate of 30% to 50%. Deep vein thrombosis in the absence of pulmonary embolism is uncommon, with a reported incidence of less than 1% [19]. Early ambulation and sequential compression devices are standard for all patients undergoing surgery. Prophylactic use of subcutaneous heparin or low molecular weight heparin (LMWH) has been recommended to help prevent venous thromboembolism. The anticoagulation efficacy of LMWH as measured by antifactor-Xa activity is lessened by increasing body weight [20]; therefore, the dose of prophylactic LMWH anticoagulation requires an adjustment based on body weight in obese patients.

Scholten and colleagues [21] showed in a retrospective study that enoxaparin, 40 mg subcutaneously every 12 hours, reduced the incidence of deep vein thrombosis significantly (0.6% versus 5.4%) compared with a 30-mg subcutaneous dose every 12 hours. Merli and colleagues [22] found in a subgroup analysis of obese patients being treated for deep vein thrombosis that a 1 mg/kg dose of enoxaparin given subcutaneously every 12 hours was more effective at preventing recurrence of deep vein thrombosis than a 1.5 mg/kg subcutaneous dose once a day. Nevertheless, there are no high-quality data to set a standard for the optimal timing, duration, and dosing of LMWH for the prevention of venous thromboembolism in patients undergoing bariatric surgery. It is common for patients with a history of deep vein thrombosis or pulmonary embolism who are undergoing bariatric surgery to have a prophylactic inferior vena caval filter placed before surgery.

The diagnosis of deep vein thrombosis or pulmonary embolism should be suspected in any patient with chest pain, shortness of breath, hypoxia, and new-onset atrial fibrillation postoperatively. Pulmonary embolism can occur immediately postoperatively before discharge and also within the first 2 months postoperatively. Diagnosis can be made with a spiral CT of the chest if the patient can fit into the scanner. Occasionally, a ventilation/perfusion scan may be helpful, but if a clinician has a strong feeling that the patient had or could have had a pulmonary embolism, one should start treatment without radiologic confirmation. There are no data to support the use of subcutaneous heparin or subcutaneous LMWH for the prevention of deep vein thrombosis after discharge from the hospital in patients who have undergone bariatric procedures. Early ambulation and a return to normal or increased activity postoperatively should help prevent deep vein thrombosis after discharge.

Nutritional and metabolic complications

Common nutritional complications arise after weight loss surgery and are addressed in a separate article in this issue by Tucker and colleagues. Iron (47%), folate (35%), and vitamin B_{12} (37%) deficiencies are common causes of anemia in bypass patients [23]. Iron deficiency is especially noted in women who are menstruating. This deficiency can be treated and prevented in most patients with daily supplemental iron therapy.

Calcium is also malabsorbed like iron because the proximal duodenum is bypassed. All bypass patients should receive 1200 mg of calcium per day to prevent hypocalcemia and osteoporosis.

All bypass patients should receive a multivitamin with folate everyday for life. If a bypass patient is losing a lot of hair, zinc deficiency may be present. Thiamine deficiency can lead to limb weakness, unsteady gait, diplopia, and confusion. Wernicke's polyneuropathy is uncommon but can lead to severe permanent neurologic deficits. These symptoms can occur in the first 2 to 4 months after surgery if vitamin B_1 is not supplemented.

Protein-calorie malnutrition is uncommon after bypass surgery but can result if the patient undergoes a long-limb or distal gastric bypass. It occurs more commonly after biliopancreatic diversion with a duodenal switch. Patients who have a low serum phosphate and low serum albumin have depletion of their total body proteins. It is important to rule out a mechanical or malabsorptive cause for the poor low protein intake. A mechanical cause of nausea or vomiting should be corrected. Malabsorption may need to be treated by converting a long-limb bypass to a standard bypass. Mild protein-calorie deficiency can corrected with protein supplements.

Weight regain

Failure of weight loss after bariatric surgery is not uncommon and occurs in approximately 10% of patients after 5 years and in about 20% of patients at 10 years [24]. The cause of weight gain can be multifactorial. The two main causes of weight gain seem to be poor eating habits and dilation of the gastric pouch, which results in overeating [25]. Patients can defeat their surgery by eating liquid sweets or other high-calorie foods despite feeling full. The best weight loss results are obtained in motivated patients who remain compliant with restrictive diets and exercise programs. Frequent follow-up visits with a nutritionist, a psychologist, and support groups seem to help patients to follow postoperative lifestyle changes.

Wound complications

Development of an incisional hernia after an open bariatric procedure is common, with an incidence of 10% to 20% [26]. Wound infections and seromas are also common after open gastric surgery for morbid obesity. These large wound seromas and infections should be drained by opening up the wound only enough to drain the seroma and infection. Cultures should be taken of the fluid that drains. Large ventral hernias that develop postoperatively and that are asymptomatic should be repaired after the patient has reached maximal weight loss. If the patient has a symptomatic ventral incisional hernia, it should be repaired to prevent incarceration and strangulation of bowel. These wound complications have almost been eliminated with the laparoscopic approach to bariatric surgery. Nevertheless, port site hernias can occur after laparoscopic bariatric procedures. The incidence of trocar site hernias is about 0.7% [19]. Patients who present with localized pain near the trocar site with or without colicky pain at or around a port site may have a partial or complete bowel obstruction. Occasionally, a palpable lump will be found on physical examination. Trocar site hernias are found radiographically on an abdominal CT. Once suspected by physical examination or found radiographically, these hernias should be reduced and repaired laparoscopically in the operating room. They can be prevented with meticulous fascial closure of all trocar sites greater than 5 mm.

Trocar site wound infections occur in less than 1% of cases. These wounds should be opened and the drainage cultured. Wounds with cellulitis should be treated with antibiotics. These deep wounds may drain for weeks. It is important to keep the skin open to allow the deep space to drain and heal from the inside out.

Leaks

Enteric leaks can arise from the stomach, intestine, and from the proximal or distal anastomosis. Enteric leaks usually appear during the first 7 to 10 days postoperatively. The first signs of an enteric leak are usually tachycardia and respiratory distress [27]. Patients may or may not complain of abdominal pain after an enteric leak. Physical examination may not reveal peritonitis. If a leak is not recognized, diagnosed, and treated in an immediate fashion, patients can develop severe intra-abdominal sepsis. In patients who are rapidly deteriorating, emergent laparoscopy or laparotomy should be done to rule out a leak.

The incidence of enteric leaks range from 2% to 7%, and they remain the second most common preventable cause of death after bariatric surgery [28]. The incidence of enteric leaks seems to decrease with experience. Wittgrove and Clark [29] reported a 4% (4 in 100) leak rate in their first 100 patients but only a 1.8% (7 in 400) leak rate in their next 400 patients. The diagnosis of enteric leaks can be challenging. The presence of an enteric leak once suspected must be confirmed radiologically or in the operating room. Many surgeons test the proximal anastomosis in the operating room with air insufflation, methylene blue, or by performing an intraoperative upper endoscopy to reveal a leak during the initial procedure. If a leak is found, the anastomosis can be repaired or reinforced before leaving the operating room. Postoperatively, a water-soluble contrast swallow or CT scan can be performed to rule out a leak. Findings that suggest a postoperative anastomotic leak are extraluminal gas, extraluminal contrast material, or both [30]. Small contained leaks can be drained percutaneously, with the patient taking nothing by mouth and fed either through the bypassed stomach or by total parenteral nutrition. A repeat swallow can be performed in 7 days. If no leak is found, a liquid diet can be resumed. If a large leak is identified, the patient must be taken back to the operating room and the anastomosis repaired or revised. Gastrointestinal leaks can be difficult to recognize. If the patient's postoperative course is not going as scheduled or the patient develops persistent tachycardia and progressive tachypnea, the clinician must rule out a leak. Mortality rates have been reported to be around 10% after the development of a postoperative gastrointestinal leak [31].

Summary

Practitioners taking care of postoperative bariatric patients need to keep in mind all of the complications that this population faces to prevent unnecessary morbidity. Bariatric patients presenting postoperatively with abdominal pain, tachycardia, vomiting, tachypnea, and a sense of impending doom should be worked up aggressively to find the cause of their symptoms. Because the incidence of obesity is rising in children and adults, more patients will have surgery to help with their weight loss. Physicians caring for these patients must be able to diagnosis and treat their complications quickly and efficiently to prevent further complications.

References

[1] Shiffman ML, Sugarman HJ, Kellum JM, et al. Gallstone formation in patients with morbid obesity: relationship to body weight, weight loss and gallbladder bile cholesterol solubility. Int J Obes Relat Metab Disord 1993;17:153–8.

[2] Shiffman ML, Sugarman HJ, Kellum JM, et al. Changes in gallbladder bile composition following gallstone formation and weight reduction. Gastroenterology 1992;103:214–21.
[3] Fobi M, Lee H, Igwe D, et al. Prophylactic cholecystectomy with gastric bypass operation: incidence of gallbladder disease. Obes Surg 2002;12:350–3.
[4] Hammad GG, Ikramuddin S, Gourash WF, et al. Elective choleycystectomy during laparoscopic roux-en-y gastric bypass: is it worth the wait? Obes Surg 2003;13:76–81.
[5] Sugarman HJ, Brewer WH, Shiffman ML, et al. A multicenter, placebo-controlled, randomized, double-blind, prospective trail of prophylactic ursodiol for the prevention of gallstone formation following gastric-bypass induced rapid weight loss. Am J Surg 1995;169:91–7.
[6] Peters M, Papasavas PK, Caushaj PF, et al. Laparoscopic transgastric endoscopic retrograde cholangiopancreatography for benign common bile duct stricture after roux-en-y gastric bypass. Surg Endosc 2002;16:1106.
[7] Nguyen NT, Stevens CM, Wolfe BM. Incidence and outcome of anastomotic stricture after laparoscopic gastric bypass. J Gastrointest Surg 2003;7:997–1003.
[8] Sapala JA, Wood MH, Sapala MA, et al. Marginal ulcers following gastric bypass: a prospective 3-year study of 173 patients. Obes Surg 1998;8:505–16.
[9] Schrimer B, Erenoglu C, Miller A. Flexible endoscopy in the management of patients undergoing Roux-en-Y gastric bypass. Obes Surg 2002;12:634–8.
[10] Scopinaro N, Gianetta E, Adami GF, et al. Biliopancreatic diversion for obesity at eighteen years. Surgery 1996;119:261–8.
[11] Gumbs AA, Duffy AJ, Bell RL. Incidence and management of marginal ulceration after laparoscopic Roux-en-Y gastric bypass. Surg Obes Relat Dis 2006;2:460–3.
[12] Gould JC, Garren MJ, Starling JR. Lessons learned from the first 100 cases in a new minimally invasive bariatric program. Obes Surg 2004;14:618–25.
[13] Brolin RE, Kenler HA, Gorman JH, et al. Long-limb gastric bypass in the superobese, a prospective randomized study. Ann Surg 1992;215:387–95.
[14] Comeau E, Gagner M, Inabnet WB, et al. Symptomatic internal hernias after laparoscopic bariatric surgery. Surg Endosc 2005;19:34–49.
[15] Champion JK, Williams M. Small bowel obstruction and internal hernias after laparoscopic Roux-en-Y gastric bypass. Obes Surg 2003;13(4):596–600.
[16] Higa KD, Ho T, Boone KB, et al. Internal hernias after laparoscopic Roux-en-Y gastric bypass: incidence, treatment, and prevention. Obes Surg 2003;13:350–4.
[17] Jones KB. Biliopancreatic limb obstruction in gastric bypass at or proximal to the jejunojejunostomy: a potentially deadly, catastrophic event. Obes Surg 1996;6:485–93.
[18] Eriksson S, Backman L, Ljungstrom KG. The incidence of clinical postoperative thrombosis after gastric surgery for obesity during 16 years. Obes Surg 1997;7:332–6.
[19] Schauer PR, Ikaramuddin S, Gourash W, et al. Outcomes after laparoscopic Roux-en-y gastric bypass for morbid obesity. Ann Surg 2000;232:515–29.
[20] Frederiksen SG, Hedenbro JL, Norgren L. Enoxaparin effect depends on body weight and current doses may be inadequate in obese patients. Br J Surg 2003;90:547–8.
[21] Scholten DJ, Hoedema RM, Scholten SE. A comparison of two different prophylactic dose regimens of low molecular weight heparin in bariatric surgery. Obes Surg 2002;12:19–24.
[22] Merli G, Spiro TE, Olsson CG, et al. Enoxaparin clinical trail group: subcutaneous enoxaparin once or twice daily compared to intravenous unfractionated heparin in the treatment of venous thromboembolic disease. Ann Intern Med 2001;134:191–202.
[23] Brolin RE, Gorman JH, Gorman RC, et al. Are vitamin B-12 and folate deficiency clinically important after Roux-en-Y gastric bypass? J Gastrointest Surg 1998;2:436–42.
[24] Christou NV, Look D, Maclean LD. Weight gain after short- and long-limb gastric bypass in patients followed for longer than 10 years. Ann Surg 2006;244(5):734–40.
[25] Maclean LD, Rhode BM, Nohr CW. Late outcomes of isolated gastric bypass. Ann Surg 2000;231:524–8.
[26] Yale CE. Gastric surgery for morbid obesity: complications and long term weight control. Arch Surg 1989;124:941–7.

[27] Hamilton EC, Sims TL, Hamilton TT, et al. Clinical predictors of leak after laparoscopic roux-en-y gastric bypass for morbid obesity. Surg Endosc 2003;17:674–84.

[28] Thodiyil PA, Rogula T, Matter SG, et al. Management of complications after laparoscopic bypass. In: Inabet WB, Demaria EJ, Irkamuddin S, editors. Laparoscopic bariatric surgery. Philadelphia: Lippincott Williams and Wilkins; 2005. p. 225–37.

[29] Wittgrove AC, Clark GW. Laparoscopic gastric bypass, roux-en-y–500 patients: technique and results, with 3–60 month follow-up. Obes Surg 2000;10:233–9.

[30] Blachar A, Federle MP, Pealer KM, et al. Gastrointestinal complications of laparoscopic roux-en-y gastric bypass surgery: clinical and imaging findings. Radiology 2002;223:625–32.

[31] Marshall JS, Srivastava A, Gupta SK, et al. Roux-en-Y gastric bypass leak complications. Arch Surg 2003;138:556–8.

ELSEVIER
SAUNDERS

THE MEDICAL
CLINICS
OF NORTH AMERICA

Med Clin N Am 91 (2007) 485–497

Laparoscopic Gastric Band Complications

Jeff W. Allen, MD

Department of Surgery, University of Louisville, Louisville, KY 40292, USA

Weight loss surgery, also known as bariatric surgery, has evolved from a specialty dominated by intestinal bypasses and vertical banded gastroplasty to its current state of a specialty characterized by minimal access techniques and Centers of Excellence. Bariatric surgery has remained the only reliably effective option for significant weight loss for the morbidly obese. There is a renewed awareness by patients, referring physicians, and surgeons in the field, and interest in bariatric surgery is at an all-time high. From 1993 to 1997, the number of weight loss operations performed in the United States increased modestly from 9189 to 12,541, but there was an increase of 450% between 1998 (12,775) and 2002 (70,256) [1,2].

In addition to the increasing rate of morbid obesity, two significant factors have contributed to the rapid increase in the number of procedures performed. The first is the advent of the laparoscopic approach to bariatric surgery. Laparoscopy carries with it the benefits of superior cosmesis, less chance of wound infection or incisional hernia, shorter hospitalization, less pain, and speedier recovery. The second factor was the approval by the Federal Drug Administration of the Lap Band System (Inamed Health, Santa Barbara, CA).

Description of the band

The Lap Band System is the only laparoscopic adjustable gastric band (LAGB) that is approved for widespread use in the United States. The silicone device has an inflatable inner surface. It is positioned just below the gastroesophageal junction and secured with sutures. Failure of these sutures can lead to a complication known as gastric prolapse or a "slip." The band is attached to an adjustment port by way of silicone tubing. The adjustment

E-mail address: jeffa@iglou.com

port is secured to the anterior abdominal wall fascia. As the patient loses weight, intraabdominal adipose tissue decreases, and the band loosens and needs to be periodically tightened. Tightening the band is accomplished by accessing the port with a non-coring Huber type needle and injecting saline solution. The inflation capacity for the three sizes of Lap Band Systems ranges from 4 to 10 ml (Table 1).

The future trend is for bariatric operations to be performed at Centers of Excellence, endorsed by the American College of Surgeons or the Surgical Review Corporation of the American Society of Bariatric Surgery. These centers have an established record of good technique, a comprehensive team approach, acceptable outcomes, and the experience to treat untoward events that can occur with these procedures. As the number of weight loss surgeries performed continues to increase, the number of patients who have complications will inevitably rise. Primary care providers are well suited to help identify and refer patients who have had bariatric surgery and are experiencing signs and symptoms of possible complications. This article reviews common problems occurring after LAGB with emphasis on conservative diagnosis and effective treatment.

Gastric band complications

Gastric prolapse

One unexpected event that can occur after a LAGB has been placed is gastric prolapse, also known as a "slip" or "slipped band." This occurs when some portion of the stomach below the band abnormally migrates up through the device. Because it is the most mobile part, the greater curve is the most commonly involved area of the stomach that comes up through the band. Gastric prolapse is the most common intra-abdominal complication after LAGB.

There are a number of mechanisms that have been proposed to cause the complication of gastric prolapse after LAGB. A failure of the plicating sutures placed to prevent gastric prolapse, for example, causes the mobile stomach to herniate up through the band. These sutures can pull through, dissolve, or break. Physical stress on the sutures, such as that caused by vomiting, can contribute to their breakage. As such, noncompliant patient behavior, such as overeating to the point of emesis, can cause a gastric prolapse.

Table 1
Balloon capacity of different sizes of lap band system of table Z

Size	Volume
9.75	4 ml
10	4 ml
VG	10 ml

The symptoms of gastric prolapse include nausea, vomiting, dysphagia, and heartburn, especially nocturnal reflux (Box 1). These symptoms are often indistinguishable from those seen when the band is adjusted too tightly or with gastroesophageal dilation. To help differentiate these clinical scenarios, one may deflate the LAGB. This procedure may be done in the office and includes preparing the skin with alcohol or povidone-iodine, palpation of the subcutaneous adjustment port, and access of the port with a noncoring Huber type needle. Aspiration of the fluid into a syringe completes the maneuver. Many bariatric surgeons exclusively perform adjustments, whereas others use primary care providers, interventional radiologists (who use fluoroscopic localization techniques for the port), or physician extenders to inject and remove the saline solution from the LAGB.

A patient who has the symptoms of caused by an LAGB being too tight or who has a suspected gastric prolapse first should undergo partial or complete deflation of the band. Nonimprovement with complete LAGB deflation strongly suggests gastric prolapse or pouch dilation and warrants radiologic or endoscopic evaluation. An upper gastrointestinal (UGI) radiograph with barium or water-soluble contrast material is the most commonly used diagnostic test to detect gastric prolapse. The UGI should be compared with radiographs taken immediately postoperatively, if they are available. A normal postoperative radiograph is characterized by the band pointing directly to the patient's left shoulder, no obstruction to flow of the contrast, and no redundant stomach above the band (Fig. 1). The UGI in the case of gastric prolapse has some degree of obstruction to flow, an excessive amount of pouch above the band, a device that points to the patient's left hip instead of left shoulder, and evidence fundus overhanging the band ("wave sign") (Fig. 2).

The acuity of treatment of a patient with gastric prolapse varies with the situation. Some patients have a chronic course with some improvement with removal of fluid. Others are more acute, with an identifiable event or time when symptoms began. The addition of abdominal pain to the other symptoms of gastric prolapse may be indicative of ischemia or necrosis of the

---

Box 1. Symptoms of Gastric Prolapse, Pouch Dilation, or a LAGB that is too Tight

Heartburn
Nocturnal reflux
Aspiration
Nausea
Vomiting
Intolerance of solids
Dysphagia

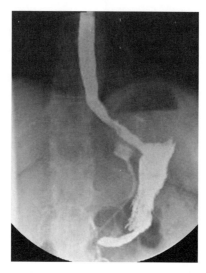

Fig. 1. Normal upper gastrointestinal radiograph after gastric band.

herniated stomach and warrants urgent therapy. Pain out of proportion to physical findings is especially concerning.

Treatment of acute gastric prolapse includes admission to the hospital, fluid resuscitation, and correction of electrolytes. Definitive therapy is operative and is usually completed using the laparoscopic approach [3]. After deflation of the device and correction of any electrolyte abnormalities, the surgeon performs exploratory laparoscopy and evaluation of the band. A nasogastric tube is placed to decompress the herniated stomach and pouch above the band.

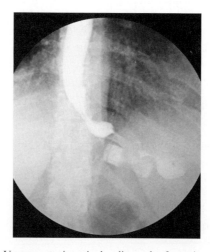

Fig. 2. Upper gastrointestinal radiograph of gastric prolapse.

Some surgeons remove and replace the band, whereas others completely take down the now scarred securing fundoplication and attempt manual reduction of the herniated portion of the stomach. If manual reduction is not successful, the surgeon may try to open the band, although this is a difficult maneuver. If the surgeon is unable to open the band or manually reduce the herniated fundus, the band may be sharply transected and replaced with a new device through a new retrogastric tunnel above the gastric prolapse.

A surgeon who is not familiar with treating this complication may opt to treat the patient by laparoscopic removal of the band. This treatment eliminates the problem of the gastric prolapse and its associated symptoms but may not be well received by the patient.

Although symptomatic improvement is an important reason to correct a gastric prolapse, there is a risk of ischemia of the herniated portion or the stomach if left untreated. Ischemia of the pouch can lead to perforation, sepsis, and death [4]. The potential lethal sequela of a prolapse is the reason why a radical approach such as band removal is occasionally chosen when this complication occurs. Band removal is likely to be unpopular with patients because not only will they need another surgery to replace the band, but they will also need insurance approval for this second operation. This "precertification" may be difficult if the patient has lost enough weight so that they are lighter than the generally accepted standards (body mass index > 40 kg/m^2) for bariatric surgery.

Gastroesophageal dilation

In many ways, the complication of gastroesophageal dilation is similar to gastric prolapse. The symptoms are not unlike those of gastric prolapse and a band adjusted too tightly, including nocturnal reflux, heartburn, dysphagia, and vomiting. Diagnosis is usually made by upper UGI, endoscopy, or diagnostic laparoscopy. Radiologic findings of gastroesophageal dilation include some obstruction to flow, an enlarged gastric pouch above the band, and an abnormally flat orientation of the band (appears transverse) (Fig. 3).

Dilation after LAGB may involve the stomach, the esophagus, or both and is felt to be due most commonly to the effects of over tightening of the band. Causative factors include an initial placement erroneously too low or too tight. In some cases, none of these factors is known to be present, and the phenomenon of dilation is considered to be idiopathic.

Management of gastroesophageal dilation is deflation of the band and observation over a period of weeks. If no immediate relief is obtained by complete deflation of the band, a surgical exploration is warranted. In most patients, the dilation resolves within 6 weeks. If UGI shows resolution of the dilation, the patient may again begin to be adjusted, although a slower, more cautious approach with more frequent, smaller adjustments is recommended. Patients who do not respond radiographically and symptomatically to LAGB deflation need operative treatment with repositioning

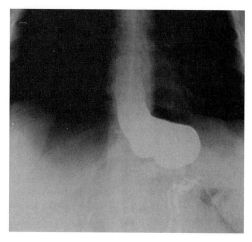

Fig. 3. Upper gastrointestinal radiograph of gastroesophageal dilation.

or removal, or consideration should be given to conversion to gastric bypass.

Band too tight

The presenting symptoms of a LAGB that is adjusted too tightly—gastric prolapse and gastroesophageal dilation—are similar and often indistinguishable. They include nausea, vomiting, intolerance of oral intake, heartburn, nocturnal regurgitation, and mild abdominal discomfort. The timing of the appearance of these symptoms is a significant factor in attempting to differentiate between a band adjusted too tightly and a gastric prolapse or gastroesophageal dilation. Symptoms that manifest within a few days of an adjustment to the band (adding fluid) are usually due to overtightening. A patient complaining of these should be seen in the office or emergency room for fluid removal and assessment.

In some instances, a band is too tight without gastroesophageal dilation or gastric prolapse. In these cases, the diagnosis of over tight band is made, and it usually follows a recent tightening of the LAGB. When this is a delayed phenomenon, the pathophysiology is less clear. It is likely that the device is borderline too tight just after the adjustment, but the patient accommodates for a short period of time, perhaps existing on liquids and slushy foods. At some point a more regular diet is attempted, and a piece of solid food becomes lodged in the stomach above the band at the narrowed portion caused by the device. On most occasions, the patient is able to expel the stuck item by self-induced forceful regurgitating. After expulsion of the object, there is edema at the gastroesophageal junction. This causes progressive dysphagia of slushy and ultimately liquid items, and soon these too can get stuck. A vicious circle follows, and the patient becomes completely obstructed. This situation can be remedied by removal of fluid. If the obstruction is long standing, there may be dehydration, and the patient may require intravenous fluids or brief admission to the hospital.

Food stuck

In unusual cases, the offending food bolus is unable to be regurgitated and does not pass with LAGB deflation. In this scenario, endoscopic retrieval may be necessary. During upper endoscopic evaluation, the obstruction may be pushed forward, or it may be retrieved per os. With the latter technique, it is important to protect the airway during retrieval.

Loosening the band

A patient who is suspected of having a band that is too tight should have fluid removed. Although there are differing techniques for tightening the band, which may include calibration with a barium meal, the removal of the fluid in a "too tight" situation is straightforward. Using sterile technique, a Huber needle is inserted into the adjustment port that is generally located on the anterior abdominal wall. The fluid is under some pressure and effluxes into the syringe readily. The patient is allowed to drink a glass of water after the deflation to ensure that the band has been loosened enough. The appropriate amount of fluid to remove from the band is difficult to know, but a good rule of thumb is to remove the amount of the last two adjustments if these are known. Complete deflation is effective but is often followed by a rapid weight gain. If the adjustment port is not easily palpable, fluoroscopic guidance can help in its localization. In some centers, physician extenders, emergency room physicians, or radiologists are trained in inflation and deflation of the LAGB, and they can be useful resources.

Erosion of the band

The gravest complication of LAGB is the erosion of the device through the gastric walls and into the lumen of the stomach. This is an unusual problem that decreases with surgeon experience. The etiology is unclear, but serosal injury at the time of placement plays a role. Additional factors may include covering the buckle with the fundoplication, subclinical chronic infection, and patient noncompliance in the form of repetitive patterns of overeating to the point of vomiting.

An eroded LAGB usually presents with vague, chronic symptoms or is asymptomatic and discovered incidentally at upper endoscopy. The most telltale sign is evidence of an infection of the adjustment port. This is due to tracking of the bacteria from inside the stomach onto the eroded band and down into the subcutaneous tissues. In addition to the port site infection, there can be occasional vague mild abdominal pain or malaise. Some patients gain weight due to the elimination of restriction of food intake because the band is longer, compressing the outside of the stomach. Infrequently, the initial presentation may be acute peritonitis; in this scenario, urgent surgical exploration is performed.

Because a patient with an eroded band usually has an adjustment port site infection, any patient who has such an infection should be evaluated for an erosion. An upper GI is usually not diagnostic of an eroded band, and the test of choice is upper endoscopy with retroflexion of the scope to visualize the potentially eroded segment just below the gastroesophageal junction. The eroded portion of the band may be the size of a pinhole. There is no evidence that any erosion, even a small one, will heal on its own.

The treatment of choice of an eroded LAGB is band removal. Sometimes there is an obvious gastrotomy around the band, and closure of this is necessary. Often the stomach has sealed the hole, and removal of the device is sufficient. The surgeon should entertain the idea of feeding jejunostomy and decompression gastrostomy tubes depending on the extent of the erosion and the overall acute and chronic health of the patient. These procedures associated with band removal usually may be accomplished laparoscopically, although the operation is often difficult due to the inflammatory reaction caused by the eroded band.

Port problems

Although problems with the adjustment port are generally neither urgent nor life threatening, they represent a significant source of morbidity for postoperative LAGB patients [5]. The adjustment port is placed in a variety of positions, based on surgeon preference, but usually resides on the anterior abdominal wall deep to the skin and superficial to the rectus sheath. Problems with the adjustment ports fall into one of four basic categories: pain, infection, leakage, or inaccessibility. Infections of the adjustment port can be early (ie, postoperative) or late, and the distinction is important with these because the etiology and treatment are different.

Because they are placed in an unnatural location, pain at the adjustment port is not completely unexpected. Usually the pain is minimal and self-limited. On occasion, the pain may be severe. Because the adjustment port is often placed in the right upper quadrant location, it is important to distinguish this from cholelithiasis by history and possibly sonographic evaluation. Persistent pain at the port should be treated by sterile local injections of a long-acting anesthetic agent around the port. If the symptoms improve but recur after the medication effect dissipates, the port should be moved surgically because it is likely entrapping a subcutaneous nerve.

An inaccessible port may be due to a thick abdominal wall over the port and may not necessarily represent a surgical problem. The patient should undergo a fluoroscopic localized adjustment to determine whether the port has flipped over. A port that is flipped 180° has an identical appearance to a port in the proper position. To differentiate between the two, the needle is passed while being visualized fluoroscopically.

A port that has flipped should be repositioned. This is likely due to one of the adjustment port anchoring sutures detaching from the fascia. Inaccessible ports need to be repositioned. The process of surgical revision includes using the previous incision and cutting down on the port. The previous sutures are removed, and the anterior rectus fascia is positively identified. The port is sutured to the fascia with four permanent sutures. A patient who is adjusted too tightly and has an inaccessible port represents an urgent situation; in such a case, the band can be deflated during the operation.

An infected adjustment port that occurs well outside the perioperative timeframe is an erosion until proven otherwise. An immediate postoperative infection at the adjustment port should be treated with oral antibiotics. Most patients respond, but some require long-term intravenous antibiotics. Occasionally, a recalcitrant infection requires adjustment port removal. In such a case, the wound is allowed to heal secondarily, and the adjustment port is replaced at a different location.

A leak in the system most commonly occurs at the port. This may be caused by a needle hitting the tubing instead of the port or by a break in the tubing due to shear force. With each adjustment, the physician should remove the saline solution in the band to ensure that there is no leakage. This is generally going to be an "all or none" phenomenon. In other words, if there is slightly less fluid within the band than anticipated, this is likely due to a measuring error and not a leak. Conversely, an empty band that has been previously adjusted successfully is a leak until proven otherwise.

Injection of water-soluble contrast material may help to identify the location of the leak. Many surgeons skip this step because it does not change the operative plan, which is replacement of the leaky portion. The operative strategy includes general anesthesia, cutting down directly on the adjustment port, identifying the leaky area by injection, and replacement. In most instances, the port alone may be replaced. On occasion, the source of the leak is not identifiable in the subcutaneous area; in such a case, the laparoscope should be used to track the source up to the band. A needle stick of the band (eg, due to a stray pass during fundal plication) is the most likely intra-abdominal culprit. Table 2 summarizes common complications and their approximate frequency.

Postoperative obstruction

With the introduction of larger bands, the complication of immediate postoperative obstruction is becoming less common. Symptoms that occur immediately after surgery include dysphagia, chest pain, vomiting, and, in some patients, intolerance of their own saliva. Diagnosis is confirmed when UGI reveals no gastric prolapse but complete or near-complete obstruction of flow of the contrast.

Table 2
Common complications of gastric banding and estimated incidence

Complication	Estimated incidence
Gastric prolapse (aka slip)	5%–10%, decreases with surgeon experience and use of pars flaccid approach
Gastroesophageal dilation	5%–10%, often due to overtightening of the band; may decrease with fluoroscopically calibrated adjustments
Band erosion	0%–2%, likely due to trauma at time of initial placement; decreases with surgeon experience
Inaccessible port	2%–5%, due to adjustment port migration or flip
Pain at adjustment port site	1%–2%, may require relocating the port
Vitamin deficiency	<1%, unusual because the operation has no malabsorptive properties
Leaking port	5%, usually due to needle stick at the adjustment port

Treatment of immediate postoperative obstruction after LAGB includes intravenous fluids and systemic anti-inflammatories, such as steroids or ketorolac. The patient is allowed to drink water as the symptoms improve but is kept nil by mouth until then. Most patients do not need operative treatment, and the obstruction improves and resolves as the postoperative edema dissipates. Reoperation is reserved for patients who do not resolve, for patients who do not tolerate the situation, and for patients in whom a clinical change that suggests perforation or ischemia. For patients who undergo surgery, strategies include band removal, exchange for a larger band, or paring down the fat inside the band.

Cholelithiasis

One of the risk factors for the development of gallstones is weight loss, especially in rapid fashion. Postoperative LAGB patients should be evaluated for signs and symptoms associated with cholelithiasis or cholecystitis. In a recent Australian study, over 800 LAGB patients without gallstones on preoperative ultrasound were followed for a median of 48 months, and 55 (6.8%) patients later presented with proven symptomatic cholelithiasis [6]. The most frequent complaint is right upper quadrant abdominal pain, especially after eating. Nausea and dyspepsia may also be present. Diagnosis is most effectively made by abdominal ultrasound. Occasionally, CT may detect gallstones. Treatment is cholecystectomy. There is usually no reason for LAGB removal, even in the face of cholecystitis, although a severe case with pancreatitis, hemodynamic instability, peritonitis, or necrosis of the gallbladder may be the exception to the rule.

Inadequate weight loss

A certain percentage of patients undergoing any weight loss operation fail, and the LAGB is no exception. The pattern of failure may be different, however. Patients who have inadequate weight loss after gastric bypass, for example, often lose the desired weight and then regain the weight. LAGB patients who struggle may do so initially, especially with an inadequate adjustment technique or schedule.

The first thing to consider in a patient who is not loosing an acceptable amount of weight is that there is a failure of the device or the adjustments. Access the port with a sterile noncoring Huber needle and determine the amount of fluid within the band. If there is no fluid in the band, there is a leak in the system, or the adjustments have missed their mark. To differentiate the two, add some fluid to the band and repeat the withdrawal procedure in a week. An empty band means a leak, and the patient should be operated upon as previously described.

If there is no leak in the system, the patient should maintain a diet log, which should be reviewed on a routine basis. Review of the log frequently demonstrates sources of noncompliance with the prescribed diet. In addition, one should consider if a band adjustment is needed. Fig. 4 is an algorithm that can be used to judge if a band is optimally adjusted. The technical exercise of band adjustment can be easily learned. Experience is needed to understand when and how much of an adjustment is needed.

Excessive weight loss

One of the benefits of the LAGB is its ability to be adjusted. This is most commonly used when patients have decelerated or plateaued weight loss. In such a case, the band is inflated. Some patients have too much weight loss, and for this problem the band is loosened. A small portion of patients have continued weight loss despite complete emptying of the band. This is proposed to be due to the decrease in hunger associated with LAGB placement or the psychologic effect of the device. In this scenario, the patient is counseled about extreme weight loss, proper diet, and realistic expectations. If this proves unsuccessful, consideration must be given to band removal. Some "triggers" for band removal include hypoalbuminemia, complications of malnutrition (eg, night blindness due to vitamin deficiency), anemia requiring multiple transfusions, and loss of over 110% excess body weight.

LAGB removal is a reasonably straightforward process and is usually accomplished laparoscopically. Patients must be educated about the possibilities of rapid weight regain after device removal and should continue to be followed because often one eating disorder (morbid obesity) is exchanged for another (bulimia or anorexia nervosa).

Summary

The LAGB is a promising new surgical therapy for the treatment of morbid obesity. Advantages over current operative modalities include an excellent safety profile, relatively easy reversibility, and adjustability. There

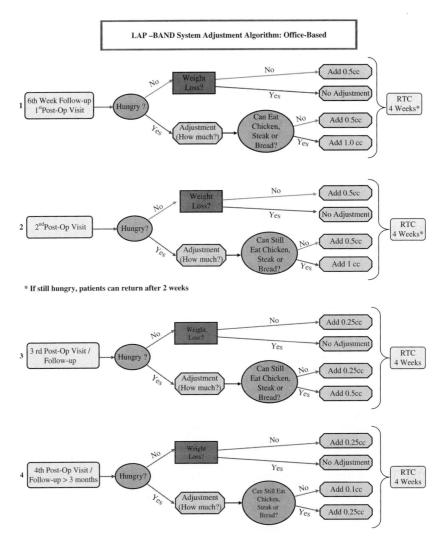

Fig. 4. LAP-BAND system adjustment algorithm: office-based. (*Courtesy of* Christine Ren, MD, New York, NY.)

are certain complications that are unique to this operation. They include gastric prolapse, gastroesophageal dilation, adjustment port problems, and erosions.

Patients who have gastroesophageal reflux and dysphagia should be evaluated for gastric prolapse, gastroesophageal prolapse, a food bolus causing an obstruction, and a band adjusted too tightly. Differentiation is made by taking a careful history and evaluating a contrast study of the esophagus and stomach. Treatment is operative in the case of the gastric prolapse,

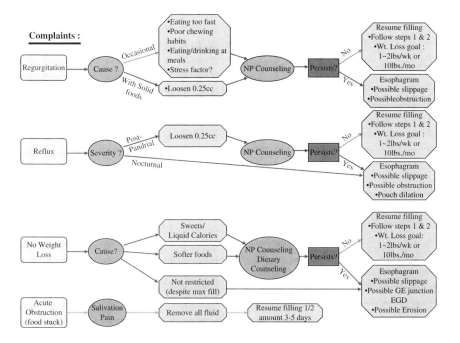

Fig. 4 (*continued*)

and usually the LAGB is repositioned or removed and replaced. Deflation of the band can improve symptoms associated with dilation and a band adjusted too tightly. Patients who do not improve should undergo upper endoscopy to evaluate for an obstruction caused by a food bolus.

Erosions and problems with the adjustment port can also occur. A LAGB that migrates inside the lumen of the stomach frequently presents with infection of the adjustment port and requires prompt removal. Adjustment ports may need to be revised or replaced due to inaccessibility, pain, or infection.

References

[1] Pope GD, Birkmeyer JP, Finlayson SR. National trends in utilization and in hospital outcomes of bariatric surgery. J Gastrointest Surg 2002;6:855–61.
[2] Nguyen NT, Root J, Kambiz Z, et al. Accelerated growth of bariatric surgery with the introduction of minimally invasive surgery. Arch Surg 2005;140:1198–202.
[3] Tran D, Rhoden DH, Cacchione RN, et al. Techniques for repair of gastric prolapse after laparoscopic gastric banding. J Laparoendosc Adv Surg Tech A 2004;14(2):117–20.
[4] Favretti F, Cadiere GB, Segato G, et al. Laparoscopic banding: selection and technique in 830 patients. Obes Surg 2002;12(3):385–90.
[5] Susmallian S, Ezri T, Elois M, et al. Access-port complications after laparoscopic gastric banding. Obes Surg 2003;13(1):128–31.
[6] O'Brien PE, Dixon JB. A rational approach to cholelithiasis in bariatric surgery: its application to the laparoscopically placed adjustable band. Arch Surg 2003;138:908–12.

ELSEVIER
SAUNDERS

THE MEDICAL
CLINICS
OF NORTH AMERICA

Med Clin N Am 91 (2007) 499–514

Nutritional Consequences
of Weight-Loss Surgery

Olga N. Tucker, MD, FRCSI,
Samuel Szomstein, MD, FACS,
Raul J. Rosenthal, MD, FACS*

*The Bariatric Institute, Cleveland Clinic Florida, 2950 Cleveland Clinic Boulevard,
Weston, FL 33331, USA*

Malnutrition is defined as "any disorder of nutrition status including disorders resulting from a deficiency of nutrient intake, impaired nutrient metabolism, or overnutrition" [1]. Overnutrition results in obesity; therefore, obesity is a form of malnutrition. The incidence of obesity is increasing at an alarming rate. Worldwide, an estimated 1.7 billion people are overweight, with an excess of 97 million obese adults in the United States [2,3]. Obesity is also a growing problem in children, and its prevalence parallels that of adult obesity [4,5].

Weight loss in obese individuals followed by long-term maintenance of an ideal weight is difficult. Increased physical activity and caloric reduction with low-calorie or low-carbohydrate diets can reduce weight by 5% to 10% over a 6-month period, but weight regain is common [6–9]. Currently available pharmacologic therapies can be combined with dietary measures for a greater weight loss effect but dose-dependent side effects limit their use, and long-term safety and efficacy beyond 2 years have not been fully evaluated [10–12]. Surgery has been demonstrated to be the most effective treatment for weight loss and improvement in some comorbid conditions in patients with morbid obesity [13,14]. Surgical approaches to induce weight loss include the use of restriction, in which food intake is limited by a small gastric pouch or reservoir, the use of malabsorption, in which the length of intestine available for nutrient absorption is reduced, or by a combination of both techniques (Box 1). Currently, laparoscopic Roux-en-Y gastric bypass (LRYGB) and laparoscopic adjustable gastric banding

* Corresponding author.
E-mail address: rosentr@ccf.org (R.J. Rosenthal).

0025-7125/07/$ - see front matter © 2007 Elsevier Inc. All rights reserved.
doi:10.1016/j.mcna.2007.01.006   *medical.theclinics.com*

500

TUCKER et al

Box 1. Surgical procedures categorized by mechanism of action

Purely restrictive
Vertical banded gastroplasty
Adjustable gastric banding
Sleeve gastrectomy
Intragastric balloon[a]

Purely malabsorptive
Jejunoileal bypass[b]
Jejunocolonic bypass[b]

Appetite suppression
Implantable gastric stimulator[c]

Malabsorption > restriction
Biliopancreatic diversion
Biliopancreatic diversion with duodenal switch
Very long limb Roux-en-Y gastric bypass

Restriction > malabsorption
Roux-en-Y gastric bypass

---

[a] Not approved for use in the United States.
[b] Abandoned techniques.
[c] Not currently available for clinical use.

(LAGB) are the most commonly performed procedures in the United States. Although surgical strategies are more successful in achieving and maintaining weight loss, nutritional deficiencies with metabolic consequences can result in the short and long term [15,16]. The severity of the postoperative nutritional deficit is dependent on several factors, including the preoperative nutritional status, the type of bariatric procedure performed, the occurrence of postoperative complications, the ability to modify eating behavior, and compliance with regular follow-up and prescribed vitamin and mineral supplementation.

Absorption of micronutrients and macronutrients in the normal gastrointestinal tract

Macronutrients

Protein metabolism
When food enters the mouth, cephalic stimulation with acetylcholine release enhances acid production from gastric parietal cells [17]. Acid and acetylcholine stimulate release of chief cell pepsinogen. Pepsinogen is cleaved to

pepsin at a pH of 5 or less, and pepsin cleaves protein to peptides. Passage of peptides and amino acids into the duodenum stimulates duodenal and jejunal epithelial cells to release cholecystokinin (CCK). Food in the antrum, antral distention, and vagal stimulation increase gastrin production, and gastrin further enhances CCK release. CCK stimulates release of pancreatic acinar cell trypsinogen, which is cleaved in the duodenum by duodenal enterokinase into its active form, trypsin. Trypsin then activates pancreatic acinar cell chymotrypsin and procarboxypeptidases A and B, which hydrolyze proteins into oligopeptides and amino acids. Oligopeptides are digested by brush border peptidases and then absorbed through the sodium-dependent amino acid cotransporters located along the luminal border of the duodenal enterocyte. Fifty percent of protein absorption occurs in the duodenum, and, by the midjejunum, the majority of protein absorption is complete [17].

Carbohydrate metabolism

Salivary and pancreatic amylase hydrolyze polysaccharides into oligosaccharides. Oligosaccharides are broken down by intestinal brush border oligosaccharidases including sucrase, maltase, and lactase to the monosaccharides glucose, fructose, and galactose [17]. Glucose and galactose are actively transported into the enterocyte by a Na+ K+ ATPase pump, while fructose is transported passively through carrier-facilitated diffusion. Carbohydrate absorption begins in the duodenum and is complete within the first 100 cm of the small intestine [17].

Lipid metabolism

Dietary lipids include free fatty acids, triglycerides, phospholipids, and cholesterol. Lipids enter the duodenum and stimulate duodenal mucosal I and S cells to secrete CCK and secretin, respectively, which stimulates gallbladder contraction and pancreatic secretion of lipase, cholesterol esterase, and phospholipase A2 to create lipid by-products [17]. Bile salts emulsify the lipid by-products in bile salt–formed micelles for transport into the enterocyte. Triglycerides and cholesterol are resynthesized within the enterocyte and combine with other nonpolar lipids, phospholipids, and proteins to form chylomicrons. From the enterocyte, chylomicrons are transported into the lymphatic system. Although 93% of dietary lipids are absorbed in the proximal two thirds of the jejunum, fat absorption, including the fat-soluble vitamins A, D, E, and K, can occur throughout the length of the small intestine. Excess bile salts are absorbed in the terminal ileum [17].

Micronutrients, vitamins, essential minerals

Fat-soluble vitamins

The fat-soluble vitamins, A, D, E, and K, diffuse across the brush border plasma membrane of the intestinal epithelial cell inside micelles formed by bile salts and lipid digestion products [17]. Although most fat-soluble vitamin absorption occurs in the proximal two thirds of the jejunum, absorption can occur throughout the small intestine. Deficiencies can occur due to reduced intake or malabsorption. In malabsorptive procedures performed for weight loss, the duodenum and varying lengths of jejunum are bypassed with resultant inadequate mixing of food with biliary and pancreatic secretions, causing steatorrhea, bile salt wasting, and malabsorption of fat-soluble vitamins.

Water-soluble vitamins

Water-soluble vitamins include B_1 (thiamine), B_2 (riboflavin), B_3 (niacin), biotin, pantothenic acid, B_6, B_{12} (cobalamin), folate, and vitamin C (ascorbate). Most water-soluble vitamins can be absorbed by simple diffusion if taken in sufficiently high doses with the exception of vitamin B_{12}. Absorption mainly occurs in the proximal small bowel, mainly in the jejunum.

Vitamin B_{12}

Cobalamin-containing foods such as meat, eggs, and milk undergo acid and peptic hydrolysis in the stomach to release vitamin B_{12}. Once liberated, vitamin B_{12} is avidly bound to glycoproteins known as R binders that are secreted in saliva, gastric juice, bile, and intestinal secretions. In the duodenum, pancreatic lipases degrade R binders and allow vitamin B_{12} to bind with intrinsic factors produced by gastric parietal cells. The intrinsic factor–vitamin B_{12} complex is bound to specific receptors in the terminal ileum and absorbed. The parietal cells that secrete acid and intrinsic factor and the chief cells that secrete pepsinogen are located primarily in the fundus and body of the stomach. Surgical procedures that produce restriction by creation of a small gastric pouch, such as RYGB, can cause significant vitamin B_{12} deficiency by reduction of acid and pepsin digestion of protein-bound cobalamins in food, incomplete release of R binders, and decreased production of intrinsic factor.

Iron

Iron is liberated from heme proteins in foods of animal origin by exposure to acid and proteases in gastric juices. The low pH of the gastric acid solubilizes iron by reducing it from the ferric to the ferrous state for absorption in the duodenum and upper jejunum. After RYGB, reduced intake of organic heme iron, reduced conversion of the ferric to ferrous state, and reduced absorption can all contribute to low iron levels, especially in premenopausal women with additional menstrual losses. Tannins, phosphates, and phytates in food reduce iron absorption, whereas ascorbic acid increases it.

Folic acid

Dietary folate is present in food in the form of polyglutamates, which are hydrolyzed by intestinal brush border conjugases to monoglutamates.

Absorption occurs primarily from the proximal third of the small intestine but can occur along the entire length of the small intestine. Folate deficiency occurs with reduced dietary intake and reduced absorption.

Calcium

Calcium is absorbed primarily in the duodenum and proximal jejunum by an active saturation process mediated by vitamin D. Deficiency can occur with reduced intake of calcium- and vitamin D–containing food, reduced absorption due to bypass of the duodenum, and malabsorption of vitamin D. When a significant amount of the stomach is excluded, such as in RYGB, calcium citrate with vitamin D is the preferred preparation for replacement because it is more soluble than calcium carbonate in the absence of gastric acid production. Phytates, phosphates, and oxalates in food reduce calcium absorption.

Other nutrients

Essential minerals and trace elements (zinc, copper, cobalt, selenium, magnesium) are absorbed in the small intestine.

Preoperative nutritional status in bariatric patients

A morbidly obese patient is not a well-nourished patient. Although obese individuals have excess stores of energy in the form of fat, they may have clinical or subclinical nutritional deficiencies because of a poor diet over a prolonged period of time [18]. Most reported studies in the literature have concentrated on perioperative nutrient deficiencies before and after biliopancreatic diversion (BPD) and biliopancreatic diversion with duodenal switch (BPD-DS). In a review of nutritional deficiencies after BPD in 94 patients and BPD-DS in 76 patients, Slater and colleagues [19] reported a significant reduction in fat-soluble vitamin levels and abnormal calcium metabolism at 1 year following surgery. At 1 year, serum vitamin A levels were low in 52% of patients, vitamin K in 51%, and vitamin D in 57%. Serum zinc levels were also low in 51%, and hypocalcemia was present in 15% with secondary hyperparathyroidism in 31% [19]. None of the patients were symptomatic. The results suggested that fat-soluble vitamin deficiency, hypocalcemia, and low zinc levels were present in many of the patients before surgery.

Other studies have demonstrated similar findings [20–23]. Compston and colleagues [22] demonstrated low preoperative serum vitamin D levels in 16% of patients, and in a separate study, Bell and colleagues [23] confirmed these findings with a mean vitamin D level of 29 ng/mL in obese patients compared with 37 ng/mL in nonobese patients. Similar deficiencies have been reported in obese patients before RYGB, which persist and may worsen after surgery if unrecognized. In a prospective study by Sanchez-Hernandez and colleagues [21], improvements in vitamin D deficiency and secondary hyperparathyroidism after RYGB were seen in 42% of patients; 37% of patients maintained their preoperative levels and 20% had a further reduction. Oral vitamin D supplementation and increased sunlight exposure were recommended in the morbidly obese [21]. Preoperative bone mineral density scans demonstrated osteopenia in 15 of 230 patients in a study by Johnson and colleagues [24], with further bone loss in the first year after RYGB.

Deficiencies of other essential vitamins, minerals, and trace elements are reported. Decsi and colleagues [25] demonstrated reduced serum vitamins A and E in obese boys compared with control values. Before LAGB, Gasteyger and colleagues [26] showed low iron levels in 31% and vitamin B_{12} deficiency in 14% of their patients. At 1 year after LAGB, serum folate levels were significantly decreased [26]. Cooper and colleagues [27] also demonstrated low serum folate at 1 year following modified VBG despite low-dose multivitamin supplementation. Reduced thiamine levels are also reported, which can result in significant neurologic sequelae. Because thiamine is absent from fats, oils, and refined sugars, patients with a high carbohydrate intake derived mainly from refined sugars and milled rice are at greater risk of thiamine deficiency. The authors' group previously evaluated preoperative thiamine levels in obese patients not taking nutritional supplements, with no history of frequent alcohol consumption, other malabsorptive conditions, or previous bariatric surgery [28]. Of 303 patients, 15.5% had low preoperative thiamine levels. Female patients had lower mean preoperative thiamine levels of 2.4 μg/dL when compared with male patients (3.2 μg/dL) [28]. Deficiencies of micronutrients including vitamins A, K, C, and E, zinc, arginine, glutamine, copper, iron, essential fatty acids, bromelain, bioflavanoids, and ornithine alpha-ketoglutarate may interfere with wound healing after surgery. These findings emphasize the importance of a thorough preoperative nutritional assessment, with intervention if deficiencies exist.

Metabolic consequences of specific bariatric procedures

Restrictive procedures

Purely restrictive procedures achieve weight loss by limiting the total daily volume of food intake. Surgical options include the vertical banded gastroplasty (VBG), LAGB, or sleeve gastrectomy [29,30]. These procedures reduce the total volume and rate of food consumption. Absorption of ingested nutrients is normal because the continuity of the stomach, duodenum, and small bowel is intact. Nutritional deficiencies are uncommon unless eating habits are excessively restricted or a complication occurs. Due to a decrease in total caloric intake and selective food intolerance, particularly to meat, the ingestion of many essential nutrients, both macronutrients and micronutrients, is reduced. Due to the inability to tolerate leafy and green vegetables, folic acid deficiency is the most common nutrient deficiency encountered after restrictive procedures. Daily multivitamin and mineral supplementation is recommended. Malnutrition can result if complications occur. Vomiting is common after VBG and LAGB and can result in significant nutritional deficiencies with dehydration and electrolyte abnormalities.

Malabsorptive procedures

Purely malabsorptive procedures include the jejunoileal (JIB) and jejunocolonic bypass (JCB). Although it resulted in significant weight loss in over 70% of patients, the JIB was abandoned owing to serious metabolic consequences including intractable diarrhea, electrolyte disturbances, severe protein-calorie malnutrition, hypocalcemia, calcium oxalate stones, vitamin deficiencies, migratory polyarthralgias, and liver dysfunction progressing to cirrhosis and liver failure [31,32]. A high proportion of JIBs have now been revised to a less malabsorptive procedure or reversed. Nevertheless, patients continue to present with the metabolic consequences of severe malabsorption with metabolic bone, hepatic, and renal disease with hyperoxaluria and renal stones [33]. Significant hypovitaminosis D osteopathy, osteopenia, and hypocalcemia owing to vitamin D deficiency have been reported in a patient 32 years after JIB [34].

Combined malabsorptive and restrictive procedures

Procedures combining malabsorption and restriction include the RYGB, BPD, and BPD-DS. The RYGB is the most commonly performed bypass procedure. Weight loss occurs owing to a reduction in gastric volume with restricted intake, the dumping syndrome precipitated by ingestion of simple sugars, and a degree of malabsorption (Fig. 1). The dumping syndrome is precipitated by the ingestion of food with a high sugar or fat content and occurs in more than 75% of patients following RYGB [35]. It generally subsides 12 to 18 months after surgery. Patients can have disabling symptoms with food aversion and dehydration. Prevention involves consumption of small frequent meals, avoidance of high sugar content foods, chewing food thoroughly, eating slowly, and drinking liquids in between meals. A wide variety of pharmacologic therapies are available for patients with severe symptoms [35]. Low levels of vitamin D, calcium, vitamin B_{12}, and iron predominate after RYGB [36]. In a series of 41 patients who underwent RYGB, Johnson and colleagues [37] demonstrated a linear decrease in vitamin D with a linear increase in parathyroid hormone over time with increased roux limb length. Secondary hyperparathyroidism with elevated parathyroid hormone was seen in 58% of the patients after RYGB with normal vitamin D levels, suggesting selective calcium malabsorption [37]. Late development of metabolic bone disease with osteomalacia can occur due to vitamin D deficiency and secondary

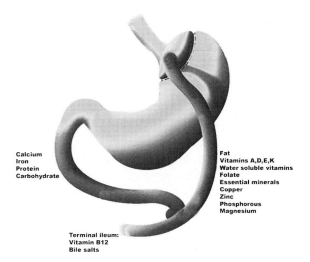

Fig. 1. Site of absorption of macronutrients and micronutrients. (*Courtesy of* the Cleveland Clinic Foundation, Cleveland, Ohio; with permission.)

hyperparathyroidism [38]. Postmenopausal women after RYGB demonstrate evidence of secondary hyperparathyroidism, elevated bone resorption, and reduced femoral neck and higher lumbar spine bone loss [39].

The BPD is primarily a malabsorptive procedure with minor restriction, consisting of a distal gastrectomy with a large 200- to 500-mL proximal pouch and a long Roux-en-Y reconstruction [40]. To reduce the adverse side effects of marginal ulceration, diarrhea, and protein-calorie malnutrition, the BPD was modified to the BPD-DS procedure [41,42]. The BPD-DS combines a vertical sleeve gastrectomy with a volume of approximately 100 to 150 mL and a duodenal switch with a common channel of 100 cm and an alimentary limb of 150 cm. Nutritional deficiencies are more common after the BPD and PBD-DS when compared with the RYGB. Fat-soluble vitamin deficiencies, protein-calorie malnutrition, hypocalcemia, diarrhea with dehydration and electrolyte disturbances, and deficiencies of zinc and selenium are common after BPD [43,44]. By retaining the pylorus, the BPD-DS procedure would be expected to reduce diarrhea and the risk of malnutrition when compared with BPD; however, in a study by Dolan and colleagues [45], similar weight loss and nutritional side effects were seen after BPD and PBD-DS, with hypoalbuminemia in 18%, anemia in 32%, hypocalcemia in 25%, and low levels of vitamins A, D, and K in nearly 50% of patients despite vitamin supplementation in over 80%.

Neurologic sequelae including encephalopathy, peripheral neuropathy, rhabdomyolysis, and Guillain-Barre syndrome have been reported following BPD and RYGB [46]. Of 957 patients in eight reports of neurologic complications after RYGB, 25% had vitamin B_{12} deficiency and 11% thiamine deficiency [46]. Vitamin A deficiency has been reported after RYGB and BPD, with ocular complications of xerophthalmia, nyctalopia, decreased visual acuity, and legal blindness [44,47].

Metabolic consequences of postoperative complications

Bariatric surgery involves an abdominal operation in a high-risk patient with significant comorbidity and the technical challenges of body habitus. None of the available surgical procedures are without complications [48–51]. Complications, whether early or late, can result in inadequate oral intake, excess gastrointestinal losses by vomiting or diarrhea, and a catabolic state with increased nutrient requirements. Early gastrointestinal complications after purely restrictive procedures are uncommon but include hemorrhage, gastric or esophageal perforation, outlet stenosis in VBG, and staple line leakage in VBG or sleeve gastrectomy. A similar range of complications can be seen after combined malabsorptive and restrictive procedures, with the addition of anastomotic leaks, fistulation, and intestinal obstruction [52]. These complications are usually detected in the immediate postoperative period and appropriate management instituted. Resultant nutritional deficiencies are rare, except in patients who have preexisting deficits. Nevertheless, acute stress and sepsis cause catabolism of lean body mass, which can be severely detrimental in an obese patient with preexisting protein depletion owing to a poor diet [53]. As is true for nonobese patients, if absence of oral intake is anticipated for 5 days or more, total parenteral nutrition or fine-bore nasojejunal feeding is recommended. These individuals are at risk for the refeeding syndrome, and serum levels of potassium, magnesium, and phosphorous should be checked daily for the first 3 days and promptly replaced if low [54].

Following recovery from the early postoperative period, other problems may arise that can contribute to nutritional deficiencies. One of the most common complaints after bariatric surgery is vomiting, occurring in 30% of patients [52]. Prolonged vomiting can result in dehydration, protein-calorie malnutrition, and thiamine deficiency resulting in neurologic sequelae [55–60]. There are multiple causes, and careful evaluation is essential (Box 2). Faintuch and colleagues [51] identified exogenous precipitating factors in 64% of 11 malnourished patients in a series of 236 patients who underwent RYGB. After VBG or LAGB, mechanical causes include outlet obstruction or stenosis, band slippage, band erosion, or cuff overdistention with LAGB [61]. Acid reflux and dysphagia are frequent accompanying symptoms contributing to inadequate oral intake. Over time, pouch and distal esophageal dilation with megaesophagus can develop.

After RYGB, stenosis of the gastrojejunostomy is a common complication occurring in 4% to 20% of patients [62–65]. Diarrhea can occur owing to food sensitivity, the dumping syndrome, lactose intolerance, malabsorption, and bacterial overgrowth and infection, causing dehydration and electrolyte

---

Box 2. Causes of vomiting after bariatric surgery

Inadequate chewing
Overdistention of the pouch by fluid
Large volume meals
Food intolerance (red meat, lactose)
Stomal outlet stenosis/obstruction
Marginal ulceration
Intestinal obstruction
Gastroesophageal reflux disease
Symptomatic gallstones
Medications
Dumping syndrome

---

imbalances. Other complications after RYGB, BPD, and BPD-DS include intestinal obstruction due to an internal, incisional, or port site hernia or adhesions (Box 3) [66,67]. Symptoms can be acute with a complete small bowel obstruction or recurrent with intermittent partial episodes of obstruction. Early intervention is important if and when complications develop to prevent ongoing symptoms. Intravenous replacement of potassium, essential vitamins including thiamine, and minerals is necessary in the presence of a history of prolonged vomiting or reduced oral intake to prevent the development of adverse nutritional and metabolic sequelae.

Modification of eating behavior

Following bariatric surgery, patients need to modify their eating behavior. After VBG, LAGB, or RYGB, patients need to reduce the food volume consumed, chew food very well, and slow the pace of eating. Failure to modify eating habits will result in vomiting and severe discomfort. The stomal size of the LAGB can be altered by filling or removing saline from the

---

Box 3. Late gastrointestinal complications after Roux-en-Y gastric bypass

Intestinal obstruction
Marginal ulcers
Stomal stenosis
Dumping syndrome
Gallstones

---

band depending on the amount of food the patient tolerates. Red meat and poultry are often not well tolerated after restrictive procedures and RYGB [68]. Failure to chew food well may result in outlet obstruction, discomfort, and vomiting. Ground or pureed meat is easier to tolerate. Fluids should not be consumed with food but taken 30 minutes before or after eating to prevent pouch filling, vomiting, or early satiety leading to grazing between meals. Each meal volume should be measured (<45 mL), each bite should be chewed 20 times, and cessation of eating should occur once the patient starts to feel full rather than waiting for the onset of discomfort. High sugar-containing drinks and sweets should be avoided to enhance weight loss. Carbonated drinks should be avoided because the carbon dioxide can lead to discomfort. Following RYGB, the ingestion of simple sugars in concentrated form will precipitate the dumping syndrome and should be omitted from the diet. Patients should be advised to avoid sugar-containing beverages, juice, concentrated sweets, and sugar-containing condiments and sauces such as sweet and sour sauce, ketchup, and certain salad dressings. High fat-containing food should be avoided, particularly after BPD and BPD-DS. Fat-free milk is advised after BPD or BPD-DS to avoid diarrhea, bloating, and excess flatulence due to lactase deficiency.

Protein-rich food should be the major component at each meal. Many studies have demonstrated reduced protein intake below recommended levels following bariatric surgery, with reduced dietary intake of iron, folate, and calcium [69]. In a retrospective review of 69 patients who had undergone RYGB 18 months to 4 years earlier by Warde-Kamar and colleagues [70], the average daily caloric intake was variable, ranging from 624 to 3486 kcal with a mean of 733 ± 630 kcal, with 44% of calories from carbohydrate, 22% from protein, and 33% from fat. Snacks accounted for 37% of the daily intake. Following VBG, patients adversely altered their diet toward soft, high-calorie food with increased intake of milk, ice cream, and solid sweets [71,72].

The role of preoperative preparation, postoperative nutrient supplementation, and surveillance

At the authors' center, before surgery, all patients are extensively assessed by a multidisciplinary team. Preoperatively, patients are encouraged to eat three meals a day, with no snacking in between. Consumption of high-protein food including meat, fish, eggs, and poultry, and avoidance of empty calorie food is advised. Physical activity is encouraged with a goal of walking for 30 minutes daily. Patients are advised to taste different protein shakes to identify their preferred preparation for postoperative use. Daily supplementation with a multivitamin with iron, vitamin B complex, and calcium is commenced after measurement of serum levels. If serum levels are low, appropriate replacement is performed.

After surgery, all patients receive multivitamin supplementation in the form of a daily multivitamin with iron, additional vitamin B_{12}, a vitamin B complex with thiamine, and vitamin C, iron, and calcium (Table 1). Zinc and biotin supplementation are optional to minimize temporary hair thinning. Additional protein should be given in the form of protein shakes. The daily requirement following RYGB is 40 to 60 g/day. Additional levels are required after BPD-DS at 60 to 90 g/day. In the authors' unit, protein shakes are administered for 2 weeks before surgery and continued for 2 to 3 weeks. Consumption of protein-rich food in the form of cheese, fish, and meat is encouraged once oral intake is established. Patients are encouraged to continue to drink protein shakes, particularly if oral intake is poor. Additional supplementation may be required in menstruating women at risk of iron deficiency anemia, during pregnancy with increased maternal and fetal requirements, and in obese adolescents [73]. Maternal malabsorption after BPD has resulted in vitamin A deficiency with development of night blindness during the third trimester of pregnancy and in vitamin A deficiency in the newborn infant [74]. The prevalence of overweight in female children and adolescents has increased from 14% in 1999 to 2000 to 16% in 2003 to 2004, with an increase in the prevalence of overweight in male

Table 1
Postoperative nutritional supplements after bariatric surgery

Nutritional supplement	RYGB	Sleeve gastrectomy	LAGB
Calcium with vitamin D	Calcium citrate, 500 mg × 3/d	Calcium citrate, 500 mg × 3/d	Calcium citrate, 500 mg × 3/d, or carbonate, 1200 mg/d
Vitamin B_{12}	Intramuscular, 1000 μg/month; oral, 100–300 μg/d; or sublingual, 500 μg/d	Oral, 100–300 μg/d; or sublingual, 500 μg/d	Not required unless low
Vitamin B complex with thiamine	1 tablet/d	1 tablet/d	1 tablet/d
Multivitamin tablet to replace	1 tablet/d	1 tablet/d	1 tablet/d
Vitamin A	1 mg/d	1 mg/d	1 mg/d
Vitamin D	5 μg/d	5 μg/d	5 μg/d
Vitamin E	100–300 mg/d	100–300 mg/d	100–300 mg/d
Vitamin K	65–80 μg/d	65–80 μg/d	65–80 μg/d
Iron	45–60 mg/d	45–60 mg/d	45–60 mg/d
Vitamin C	500 mg/d	500 mg/d	500 mg/d
Zinc	15 mg/d	15 mg/d	15 mg/d
Biotin	3000 μg/d	3000 μg/d	3000 μg/d

children and adolescents from 14% to 18% [5]. These patients require close monitoring and careful nutrient supplementation following surgery.

Following all bariatric surgical procedures, patients require regular and prolonged follow-up to assess weight loss, ensure compliance with diet and multivitamin and nutritional supplements, and monitor for the development of complications including nutritional deficiencies and electrolyte abnormalities. In the authors' center, all patients are seen in the outpatient clinic at 2 weeks and then every 3 months thereafter for the first year with the exception of the LAGB group, who are reviewed every 2 months. Patients are then seen every 6 months with the option of a shared medical appointment. Continuing patient education is critical to prevent noncompliance. Numerous studies have demonstrated poor compliance with vitamin and mineral supplements coupled with reduced dietary intake of below 50% of the recommended daily allowance [36,75,76].

Summary

Nutritional deficiencies are already present in many morbidly obese patients before surgery. Appropriate preoperative detection and correction is essential. Deficiencies in vitamins, minerals, proteins, lipids, carbohydrates, electrolytes, and trace elements can occur after all types of bariatric surgery. The severity and pattern is dependent on the presence of preoperative uncorrected deficiency, the type of procedure performed varying with the degree of restriction and the length of bypassed small intestine, the modification of eating behavior, the development of complications, compliance with oral multivitamin and mineral supplementation, and compliance with follow-up. Rigorous control of fluids and electrolytes with establishment of adequate oral nutrition is important in the immediate postoperative period. Regular follow-up of the metabolic and nutritional status of the patient is essential, with life-long multivitamin and mineral supplementation. Pregnancy should not be considered until at least 18 months after bariatric surgery following the completion of the period of rapid weight loss.

References

[1] ASPEN Board of Directors and Standards Committee. Definitions of terms, style, and conventions used in ASPEN guidelines and standards. Nutr Clin Pract 2005;20:281–5.
[2] Kuczmarski RJ, Flegal KM, Campbell SM, et al. Increasing prevalence of overweight among US adults: the National Health and Nutrition Examination Surveys, 1960 to 1991. JAMA 1994;272(3):205–11.
[3] Deitel M. The obesity epidemic. Obes Surg 2006;16(4):377–8.
[4] Inge TH, Zeller M, Garcia VF, et al. Surgical approach to adolescent obesity. Adolesc Med Clin 2004;15(3):429–53.
[5] Ogden CL, Carroll MD, Curtin LR, et al. Prevalence of overweight and obesity in the United States, 1999–2004. JAMA 2006;295(13):1549–55.

[6] Yanovski SZ, Yanovski JA. Obesity. N Engl J Med 2002;346(8):591–602.

[7] Leser MS, Yanovski SZ, Yanovski JA, et al. A low-fat intake and greater activity level are associated with lower weight regain 3 years after completing a very-low-calorie diet. J Am Diet Assoc 2002;102(9):1252–6.

[8] Solomon CG, Dluhy RG. Bariatric surgery—quick fix or long-term solution? N Engl J Med 2004;351(26):2751–3.

[9] Foster GD, Wyatt HR, Hill JO, et al. A randomized trial of a low-carbohydrate diet for obesity. N Engl J Med 2003;348(21):2082–90.

[10] Thearle M, Aronne LJ. Obesity and pharmacologic therapy. Endocrinol Metab Clin North Am 2003;32(4):1005–24.

[11] DeWald T, Khaodhiar L, Donahue MP, et al. Pharmacological and surgical treatments for obesity. Am Heart J 2006;151(3):604–24.

[12] Li Z, Maglione M, Tu W, et al. Meta-analysis: pharmacologic treatment of obesity. Ann Intern Med 2005;142(7):532–46.

[13] Maggard MA, Shugarman LR, Suttorp M, et al. Meta-analysis: surgical treatment of obesity. Ann Intern Med 2005;142(7):547–59.

[14] Gastrointestinal surgery for severe obesity. Consens Statement 1991;9(1):1–20.

[15] Alvarez-Leite JI. Nutrient deficiencies secondary to bariatric surgery. Curr Opin Clin Nutr Metab Care 2004;7(5):569–75.

[16] Mason ME, Jalagani H, Vinik AI. Metabolic complications of bariatric surgery: diagnosis and management issues. Gastroenterol Clin North Am 2005;34(1):25–33.

[17] Ponsky TA, Brody F, Pucci E. Alterations in gastrointestinal physiology after Roux-En-Y gastric bypass. J Am Coll Surg 2005;201(1):125–31.

[18] Boylan LM, Sugerman HJ, Driskell JA. Vitamin E, vitamin B-6, vitamin B-12, and folate status of gastric bypass surgery patients. J Am Diet Assoc 1988;88(5):579–85.

[19] Slater GH, Ren CJ, Siegel N, et al. Serum fat-soluble vitamin deficiency and abnormal calcium metabolism after malabsorptive bariatric surgery. J Gastrointest Surg 2004;8(1):48–55.

[20] Hamoui N, Kim K, Anthone G, et al. The significance of elevated levels of parathyroid hormone in patients with morbid obesity before and after bariatric surgery. Arch Surg 2003;138(8):891–7.

[21] Sanchez-Hernandez J, Ybarra J, Gich I, et al. Effects of bariatric surgery on Vitamin D status and secondary hyperparathyroidism: a prospective study. Obes Surg 2005;15(10):1389–95.

[22] Compston JE, Vedi S, Ledger JE, et al. Vitamin D status and bone histomorphometry in gross obesity. Am J Clin Nutr 1981;34(11):2359–63.

[23] Bell NH, Epstein S, Greene A, et al. Evidence for alteration of the vitamin D–endocrine system in obese subjects. J Clin Invest 1985;76(1):370–3.

[24] Johnson JM, Maher JW, Samuel I, et al. Effects of gastric bypass procedures on bone mineral density, calcium, parathyroid hormone, and vitamin D. J Gastrointest Surg 2005;9(8):1106–10.

[25] Decsi T, Molnar D, Koletzko B. Reduced plasma concentrations of alpha-tocopherol and beta-carotene in obese boys. J Pediatr 1997;130(4):653–5.

[26] Gasteyger C, Suter M, Calmes JM, et al. Changes in body composition, metabolic profile and nutritional status 24 months after gastric banding. Obes Surg 2006;16(3):243–50.

[27] Cooper PL, Brearley LK, Jamieson AC, et al. Nutritional consequences of modified vertical gastroplasty in obese subjects. Int J Obes Relat Metab Disord 1999;23(4):382–8.

[28] Carrodeguas L, Kaidar-Person O, Szomstein S, et al. Preoperative thiamine deficiency in obese population undergoing laparoscopic bariatric surgery. Surg Obes Relat Dis 2005;1(6):517–22.

[29] Mason EE, Doherty C, Cullen JJ, et al. Vertical gastroplasty: evolution of vertical banded gastroplasty. World J Surg 1998;22(9):919–24.

[30] Roa PE, Kaidar-Person O, Pinto D, et al. Laparoscopic sleeve gastrectomy as treatment for morbid obesity: technique and short-term outcome. Obes Surg 2006;16(10):1323–6.

[31] Brown RG, O'Leary JP, Woodward ER. Hepatic effects of jejunoileal bypass for morbid obesity. Am J Surg 1974;127(1):53–8.
[32] Moxley RT III, Pozefsky T, Lockwood DH. Protein nutrition and liver disease after jejunoileal bypass for morbid obesity. N Engl J Med 1974;290(17):921–6.
[33] Nordenvall B, Backman L, Larsson L. Oxalate metabolism after intestinal bypass operations. Scand J Gastroenterol 1981;16(3):395–9.
[34] Haria DM, Sibonga JD, Taylor HC. Hypocalcemia, hypovitaminosis d osteopathy, osteopenia, and secondary hyperparathyroidism 32 years after jejunoileal bypass. Endocr Pract 2005;11(5):335–40.
[35] Ukleja A. Dumping syndrome: pathophysiology and treatment. Nutr Clin Pract 2005;20(5): 517–25.
[36] Ledoux S, Msika S, Moussa F, et al. Comparison of nutritional consequences of conventional therapy of obesity, adjustable gastric banding, and gastric bypass. Obes Surg 2006; 16(8):1041–9.
[37] Johnson JM, Maher JW, Demaria EJ, et al. The long-term effects of gastric bypass on vitamin D metabolism. Ann Surg 2006;243(5):701–4.
[38] Collazo-Clavell ML, Jimenez A, Hodgson SF, et al. Osteomalacia after Roux-En-Y gastric bypass. Endocr Pract 2004;10(3):195–8.
[39] St George LI, Lin D. Malabsorption in pregnancy after biliopancreatic diversion for morbid obesity. Med J Aust 2005;182(6):308–9.
[40] Scopinaro N, Adami GF, Marinari GM, et al. Biliopancreatic diversion. World J Surg 1998; 22(9):936–46.
[41] Hess DS, Hess DW. Biliopancreatic diversion with a duodenal switch. Obes Surg 1998;8(3): 267–82.
[42] Marceau P, Hould FS, Simard S, et al. Biliopancreatic diversion with duodenal switch. World J Surg 1998;22(9):947–54.
[43] Newbury L, Dolan K, Hatzifotis M, et al. Calcium and vitamin D depletion and elevated parathyroid hormone following biliopancreatic diversion. Obes Surg 2003;13(6):893–5.
[44] Hatizifotis M, Dolan K, Newbury L, et al. Symptomatic vitamin A deficiency following biliopancreatic diversion. Obes Surg 2003;13(4):655–7.
[45] Dolan K, Hatzifotis M, Newbury L, et al. A clinical and nutritional comparison of biliopancreatic diversion with and without duodenal switch. Ann Surg 2004;240(1):51–6.
[46] Koffman BM, Greenfield LJ, Ali II, et al. Neurologic complications after surgery for obesity. Muscle Nerve 2006;33(2):166–76.
[47] Lee WB, Hamilton SM, Harris JP, et al. Ocular complications of hypovitaminosis A after bariatric surgery. Ophthalmology 2005;112(6):1031–4.
[48] Abell TL, Minocha A. Gastrointestinal complications of bariatric surgery: diagnosis and therapy. Am J Med Sci 2006;331(4):214–8.
[49] Papasavas PK, Caushaj PF, McCormick JT, et al. Laparoscopic management of complications following laparoscopic Roux-En-Y gastric bypass for morbid obesity. Surg Endosc 2003;17(4):610–4.
[50] Podnos YD, Jimenez JC, Wilson SE, et al. Complications after laparoscopic gastric bypass: a review of 3464 cases. Arch Surg 2003;138(9):957–61.
[51] Faintuch J, Matsuda M, Cruz ME, et al. Severe protein-calorie malnutrition after bariatric procedures. Obes Surg 2004;14(2):175–81.
[52] Ukleja A, Stone RL. Medical and gastroenterologic management of the post-bariatric surgery patient. J Clin Gastroenterol 2004;38(4):312–21.
[53] Ecklund MM. Meeting the nutritional needs of the bariatric patient in acute care. Crit Care Nurs Clin North Am 2004;16(4):495–9.
[54] Elliot K. Nutritional considerations after bariatric surgery. Crit Care Nurs Q 2003;26(2): 133–8.
[55] Mason EE. Starvation injury after gastric reduction for obesity. World J Surg 1998;22(9): 1002–7.

[56] Worden RW, Allen HM. Wernicke's encephalopathy after gastric bypass that masqueraded as acute psychosis: a case report. Curr Surg 2006;63(2):114–6.

[57] Toth C, Voll C. Wernicke's encephalopathy following gastroplasty for morbid obesity. Can J Neurol Sci 2001;28(1):89–92.

[58] Sola E, Morillas C, Garzon S, et al. Rapid onset of Wernicke's encephalopathy following gastric restrictive surgery. Obes Surg 2003;13(4):661–2.

[59] Albina JE, Stone WM, Bates M, et al. Catastrophic weight loss after vertical banded gastroplasty: malnutrition and neurologic alterations. JPEN J Parenter Enteral Nutr 1988;12(6): 619–20.

[60] Angstadt JD, Bodziner RA. Peripheral polyneuropathy from thiamine deficiency following laparoscopic Roux-en-Y gastric bypass. Obes Surg 2005;15(6):890–2.

[61] Fobi M, Lee H, Igwe D, et al. Band erosion: incidence, etiology, management and outcome after banded vertical gastric bypass. Obes Surg 2001;11(6):699–707.

[62] Carrodeguas L, Szomstein S, Zundel N, et al. Gastrojejunal anastomotic strictures following laparoscopic Roux-En-Y gastric bypass surgery: analysis of 1291 patients. Surg Obes Relat Dis 2006;2(2):92–7.

[63] Schwartz ML, Drew RL, Roiger RW, et al. Stenosis of the gastroenterostomy after laparoscopic gastric bypass. Obes Surg 2004;14(4):484–91.

[64] Ahmad J, Martin J, Ikramuddin S, et al. Endoscopic balloon dilation of gastroenteric anastomotic stricture after laparoscopic gastric bypass. Endoscopy 2003;35(9):725–8.

[65] Go MR, Muscarella P, Needleman BJ, et al. Endoscopic management of stomal stenosis after Roux-en-Y gastric bypass. Surg Endosc 2004;18(1):56–9.

[66] Cho M, Carrodeguas L, Pinto D, et al. Diagnosis and management of partial small bowel obstruction after laparoscopic antecolic antegastric Roux-en-Y gastric bypass for morbid obesity. J Am Coll Surg 2006;202(2):262–8.

[67] Nguyen NT, Huerta S, Gelfand D, et al. Bowel obstruction after laparoscopic Roux-en-Y gastric bypass. Obes Surg 2004;14(2):190–6.

[68] Balsiger BM, Kennedy FP, Abu-Lebdeh HS, et al. Prospective evaluation of Roux-en-Y gastric bypass as primary operation for medically complicated obesity. Mayo Clin Proc 2000; 75(7):673–80.

[69] Blake M, Fazio V, O'Brien P. Assessment of nutrient intake in association with weight loss after gastric restrictive procedures for morbid obesity. Aust N Z J Surg 1991;61(3):195–9.

[70] Warde-Kamar J, Rogers M, Flancbaum L, et al. Calorie intake and meal patterns up to 4 years after Roux-en-Y gastric bypass surgery. Obes Surg 2004;14(8):1070–9.

[71] Brolin RL, Robertson LB, Kenler HA, et al. Weight loss and dietary intake after vertical banded gastroplasty and Roux-en-Y gastric bypass. Ann Surg 1994;220(6):782–90.

[72] Kriwanek S, Blauensteiner W, Lebisch E, et al. Dietary changes after vertical banded gastroplasty. Obes Surg 2000;10(1):37–40.

[73] Sugerman HJ. Bariatric surgery for severe obesity. J Assoc Acad Minor Phys 2001;12(3): 129–36.

[74] Huerta S, Rogers LM, Li Z, et al. Vitamin A deficiency in a newborn resulting from maternal hypovitaminosis A after biliopancreatic diversion for the treatment of morbid obesity. Am J Clin Nutr 2002;76(2):426–9.

[75] Bloomberg RD, Fleishman A, Nalle JE, et al. Nutritional deficiencies following bariatric surgery: what have we learned? Obes Surg 2005;15(2):145–54.

[76] Trostler N, Mann A, Zilberbush N, et al. Nutrient intake following vertical banded gastroplasty or gastric bypass. Obes Surg 1995;5(4):403–10.

THE MEDICAL
CLINICS
OF NORTH AMERICA

ELSEVIER
SAUNDERS

Med Clin N Am 91 (2007) 515–528

Improvement in Infertility and Pregnancy Outcomes after Weight Loss Surgery

Jitesh A. Patel, MD[a], Joseph J. Colella, MD[b,c],
Emmanuel Esaka, MD, PhD[d],
Nilesh A. Patel, MD[e,*], Ronald L. Thomas, MD[f,g]

[a]Department of Surgery, Allegheny General Hospital,
320 East North Avenue, Pittsburgh, PA 15212, USA
[b]Department of Surgery, Drexel University College of Medicine, 2900 W. Queen Lane,
Philadelphia, PA 19129, USA
[c]Division of Bariatric Surgery, Department of Surgery, Allegheny General Hospital,
320 East North Avenue, Pittsburgh, PA 15212, USA
[d]Department of Obstetrics and Gynecology, Allegheny General Hospital,
320 East North Avenue, Pittsburgh, PA 15212, USA
[e]Department of Surgery, University of Texas Health Science Center San Antonio,
7703 Floyd Curl Drive, MC7740, San Antonio, TX 78229, USA
[f]Department of Obstetrics and Gynecology, Drexel University College of Medicine,
2900 W. Queen Lane, Philadelphia, PA 19129, USA
[g]Division of Maternal/Fetal Medicine, Department of Obstetrics and Gynecology,
Allegheny General Hospital, 320 East North Avenue, Pittsburgh, PA 15212, USA

There has been a significant increase in the worldwide prevalence of obesity over the past 20 years. Currently, 8% to 10% of American women and 5% of American men are categorized as "morbidly obese" and have a body mass index (BMI) of 40 kg/m^2 or greater [1]. To control this new epidemic, bariatric surgery has been shown to provide substantial and durable weight loss, improve the overall quality of life, and cure many obesity-associated diseases in the morbidly obese population [2]. At the 1991 National Institutes of Health Consensus Developmental Conference, it was concluded that bariatric surgery is the sole effective treatment for patients who have morbid obesity [3]. Furthermore, the Roux-en-Y gastric bypass (RYGB)

* Corresponding author. P.O. Box 691996, San Antonio, TX 78229.
  E-mail address: drpatel@bypassdoc.com (N.A. Patel).

0025-7125/07/$ - see front matter © 2007 Elsevier Inc. All rights reserved.
doi:10.1016/j.mcna.2007.01.002   *medical.theclinics.com*

procedure is considered the gold standard for weight loss surgery in the United States [4,5].

According to the National Health and Nutrition Examination Survey, there was a greater than fourfold increase in the prevalence of obesity in women 20 to 39 years of age from 1960 to 2000 [6]. Young women make up the majority of patients who undergo bariatric surgery yearly. A recent meta-analysis showed that more than 70% of these procedures are performed in women [2]. Others report that more than 80% of patients undergoing RYGB are women, with the majority of them being of child-bearing age [7,8]. Although it is has been shown that bariatric surgery provides a superior treatment for obesity, its effect on subsequent pregnancy has been questioned.

Maternal obesity introduces multiple risks to the mother and fetus during pregnancy (Box 1) [9–16]. Obesity has been shown to be an independent risk factor for adverse obstetric outcome for mother and fetus [9]. Dietary weight loss has been shown to greatly improve pregnancy outcome; the same should be true after weight loss surgery. In the initial reports studying patients who have undergone bariatric surgery before pregnancy, the prevalence of some of these obesity-related complications was decreased, but several new complications were introduced, such as severe malnutrition requiring parenteral nutrition, premature births, neural tube defects, fetal growth retardation, and spontaneous abortions [17–20]. Consequently, pregnancy after bariatric surgery has been a subject of concern among patients, primary care physicians, obstetricians, and bariatric surgeons. It was subsequently concluded that pregnancy after bariatric surgery was not safe and resulted in poor maternal and fetal outcomes [21–23].

These initial reports were based on the now abandoned jejunoileal bypass procedure and on the less commonly performed biliopancreatic diversion procedure, and have been contested as different bariatric procedures have been developed (eg, the RYGB and adjustable gastric band [AGB]

Box 1. Obesity-related complications of pregnancy

Pregnancy-induced hypertension
Gestational diabetes
Macrosomia
Excessive weight gain
Cesarean section
Preeclampsia
Postpartum hemorrhage
Congenital anomalies
Endometritis
Wound complications

procedures). More recent studies have demonstrated that pregnancy after a bariatric procedure is not only safe but may be associated with fewer risks or complications in comparison to the patient who remains obese during pregnancy. The purposes of this article are (1) to establish the safety of pregnancy after bariatric surgery, particularly in the setting of an experienced, multidisciplinary, bariatric center; (2) to make recommendations in perinatal management; (3) to discuss fertility and contraception; and (4) to discuss the management of postoperative complications in patients who have undergone bariatric surgery.

Current literature

Several recent reports have demonstrated good outcomes in pregnancies after bariatric surgery (Table 1). Included is our unpublished series of pregnancies after laparoscopic Roux-en-Y gastric bypass (LRYGB) at Allegheny General Hospital (Jitesh A. Patel, MD, unpublished data, 2007). The majority of these studies focused on the RYGB and the laparoscopic adjustable gastric band (LAGB), which are the preferred procedures in the United States and Europe, respectively. Although the experience is limited, there is a relatively low incidence of pregnancy-related complications.

The consensus of the current literature is that pregnancy should be delayed for up to 2 years after bariatric surgery. Although little evidence exists in the literature showing that pregnancy during this time interval is associated with poor outcome, this period is associated with the majority of the weight loss and postoperative complications. The postoperative catabolic state caused by the surgery results in dramatic weight loss and malnutrition. During this time, the patient's nutritional status should be closely monitored. Patients undergoing RYGB are prone to nutritional deficiencies given the procedure's partly malabsorptive mechanism of weight loss. Our patients are typically prescribed an empiric regimen of multivitamin twice a day after the procedure. Further supplementation may be elicited based upon clinical grounds or laboratory testing. In our experience, 30% to 50% of patients require further supplementation of calcium, iron, or vitamin B_{12}. Most of these deficiencies can be supplemented orally [24–26].

By the time this period of rapid weight loss has passed, most nutritional deficiencies have been identified and treated. After this period, pregnancy and delivery can be achieved safely and may be associated with outcomes superior to pregnancies previously carried by these patients or when compared with obese patients [27–37]. Our experience with pregnancies after weight loss surgery is similar to those previously published. Pregnancy after weight loss surgery has good maternal and fetal outcomes. In comparing our results with previously published reports, the rates of macrosomia, pregnancy-induced hypertension, preeclampsia, and gestational diabetes in patients who have undergone bariatric surgery are lower than those of

Table 1
Recent experience with pregnancies after weight loss surgery

Author	Procedure	Number of pregnancies	Spontaneous abortions	Cesarean deliveries	Pregnancy morbidities	Recommended interval from surgery to conception
Richards et al [35]	RYGB	57	n/a	14	Two perinatal deaths, nine macrosomia, four SGA, five mHTN, three GDM	n/a
Rand and Macgregor [34]	RYGB	21	n/a	6	Two neonatal jaundice, two SGA	12 mo
Bilenka et al [36]	VBG	14	1	n/a	Two mHTN, one pre-eclampsia, one intrauterine death	none
Wittgrove et al [32]	RYGB	49	7	13	One GDM, two macrosomia, four PTL	12–18 mo
Weiss et al [37]	LAGB	7	2	2	None	2 yr
Skull et al [27]	LAGB	49	n/a	12	Two neonatal complications, four GDM, four mHTN	n/a
Sheiner et al [30]	various	298	n/a	75	28 macrosomia, 15 congenital malformations, one perinatal death	n/a
Dixon et al [29]	LAGB	79	n/a	n/a	five pre-eclampsia, 5 GDM, eight mHTN, fivr SGA, nine macrosomia	12 mo
Bar-Zohar et al [33]	LAGB	81	0	17	Six mHTN, 13 GDM	n/a
Allegheny General Hospital	RYGB	24	0	15	Two macrosomia, one IUGR, one GDM	18–24 mo

Abbreviations: GDM, gestational diabetes; IUGR, intrauterine growth retardation; LAGB, laparoscopic adjustable gastric band; mHTN, maternal hypertension; PTL, pre-term labor; RYGB, Roux-en-Y gastric bypass; SGA, small for gestational age; VBG, vertical banded gastroplasty.

gravid obese women and are similar to those of nonobese women in the general population (Table 2) [38–40].

Nutritional management and patient follow-up

All patients undergoing RYGB at our institution are empirically prescribed a regimen of multivitamins after surgery. Once pregnancy has been established after weight loss surgery, nutritional assessments are continued primarily on clinical grounds. We typically recommend oral protein supplementation in patients who have no weight gain or weight loss regardless of BMI during pregnancy. Supplementation is also given if fetal growth falls below the 50th percentile. Empiric oral protein supplementation is instituted in patients who have become pregnant in the few months after bariatric surgery because of the anticipated rapid weight loss. With this regimen, we have noted that most patients after bariatric surgery require oral protein supplementation if they become pregnant within the first 12 months of bariatric surgery. During the interval of 12 to 18 months after surgical weight loss, most patients do not require supplementation, and beyond this interval, a need for supplementation is uncommon.

Pregnant patients are typically followed monthly until the 26th week (ie, the third trimester). Then, they are seen every 2 weeks and weekly after the 36th week. Patients who have gestational diabetes and maternal hypertension are followed more frequently. During these visits, lab work is not routinely ordered, with the exception of a complete blood count to assess for anemia. Examination of fundal height may be difficult in the obese gravida, and we tend to use ultrasound more liberally in these patients to assess fetal growth, particularly during the third trimester.

With our nutritional and follow-up regimen, we feel that neither the patient nor the physician are discouraged or burdened with excessive interventions. We feel that such a regimen allows the pregnancy to be followed without subjecting the patient or fetus to unnecessary interventions or

Table 2
Outcomes of pregnancy after laparoscopic Roux-en-Y gastric bypass compared among obese and non-obese populations

	Allegheny General Hospital (%)	Non-obese[a] (%)	Obese[a] (%)
Cesarean section	62.5	10.8–15.4	19.6–50
Macrosomia	8.3	8.4–11.6	16.8–42.3
Pregnancy-induced HTN	4.2	0.5–0.6	7.2–7.7
Pre-eclampsia	0	2.0	11.5
Gestational DM	4.2	1.8	5.4–15.4

Abbreviation: HTN, hypertension.
[a] *Data from* Refs [38–40].

expense while still providing a good outcome. In the setting of an experienced center, the superiority of a more rigorous management regimen is unfounded.

Management of the adjustable gastric band during pregnancy

The adjustable gastric band is the only accepted procedure for weight loss where the degree of gastric restriction may readily be manipulated. The band can be adjusted by the bariatric surgeon during and after pregnancy to achieve "optimal nutrition." In pregnancies complicated by severe nausea and emesis (eg, hyperemesis gravidarum), complete deflation of the gastric band may obviate the need for supplemental intravenous fluids or parenteral nutrition. The patients' concern of excessive weight gain during pregnancy is well taken; however, weight gain seems to be modest despite band adjustments [27,37]. Another advantage of this device is that the balloon is accessed through a percutaneous port; therefore, the procedure can typically be done in the office setting, and the device does not usually require the use of fluoroscopy or ultrasound to access.

A consensus for optimal band management during pregnancy does not exist. The management protocol ranges from deflating the balloon completely for symptoms of nausea and vomiting after the diagnosis of pregnancy to deflation if the patient is suffering from hyperemesis gravidarum [27,37]. The balance is between providing adequate nutrition to the fetus while controlling weight gain in the mother. Table 3 summarizes the recently

Table 3
Management of the adjustable gastric band during pregnancy

	Maternal BMI at conception (kg/m^2)	Mean maternal weight gain (kg)	Band management strategy
Skull et al [27]	32.8	3.7	18% adjusted; goal of minimal maternal weight gain; band emptied for hyperemesis gravidarum
Dixon et al [41]	35	8.3	100% adjusted; goal of optimal weight gain; band adjusted throughout pregnancy
Weiss et al [37]	34.8	BMI increased to 38.0 kg/m^2	100% adjusted; bands deflated to relieve nausea and vomiting
Bar-Zohar et al [33]	30.3	10.6	Goal of optimal weight gain

Abbreviation: BMI, body mass index.

published experience with the LAGB and various strategies in band management during pregnancy.

All four authors have different strategies in band management. Skull and colleagues [27], Bar-Zohar and colleagues [33], and Dixon and colleagues [41] reported good outcomes. These three studies demonstrated a lower prevalence of obesity-associated complications without added neonatal risks when compared with obese control subjects who had not undergone LAGB. Weiss and colleagues [37] reported that two pregnancies (29%) ended in spontaneous abortions. All of their patients had become pregnant unexpectedly within 2 years of bariatric surgery. The results of this latter study demonstrate the necessity to delay pregnancy for several months to have optimal maternal and fetal outcome.

Abdominal pain: a consequence of pregnancy or a complication of bariatric surgery?

The complaints of recurrent nausea and vomiting are common in a patient who is pregnant and after bariatric surgery. Rarely do these patients have a specific pregnancy-related or surgical complication. Initially, a thorough history, physical examination, and clinical assessment should ensue. This is important in the patient who has not been compliant with their follow-up visits with their bariatric surgeon or is several years out from their procedure. These seemingly benign symptoms may represent a chronic underlying complication from the bariatric procedure or an acute problem that may lead to fulminant peritonitis if not expeditiously assessed and treated.

The complications of bariatric surgery should not be neglected when assessing the postoperative pregnant patient. Some of the more common complications include biliary and ulcer disease. Complications such as band erosion, band slippage, and gastric prolapse are well described after vertical-banded gastroplasty and AGB [27,33,37]. Anastomotic strictures and internal hernias are seen after RYGB. Internal hernias seem to be more common with LRYGB than with RYGB [42,43]. A thorough evaluation should include a detailed history, physical examination, and basic lab work, such as a comprehensive metabolic panel and a complete blood count. When evaluating this type of patient, it is in the best interest of the mother and fetus that a bariatric surgeon be consulted early in the course of evaluation. This prevents unnecessary delays and perhaps leads to a more efficient evaluation. At our institution, all pregnant patients after weight loss surgery are routinely followed by a high-risk obstetrician and a bariatric surgeon.

Appropriate diagnostic studies may be best determined by the surgeon. Given the range of pathology, studies may include an upper gastrointestinal series, esophagoscopy, abdominal ultrasound, and CT. The difficulty with the postoperative bariatric patient, which makes early involvement of the surgeon even more critical, is that tests such as abdominal sonograms and CT scans may be inaccurate or imprecise in this patient population: Radiologic cholelithiasis is often an incidental finding, and a patient who has an internal hernia may have a CT that is interpreted as "normal" [42–45]. The current thought among many bariatric surgeons is that an exploratory laparoscopy may be the only reliable method of ruling out an internal hernia and should be performed is there is a high index of clinical suspicion [42,46]. We have a low threshold for laparoscopic exploration in the appropriate clinical setting.

Multiple reports exist of pregnant women developing peritonitis secondary to a bariatric surgery complication (Table 4). There is a wide range of surgery-to-pregnancy intervals demonstrating that these complications may present from months to years after the surgery. Although all of these cases required emergent laparotomy and many required emergent delivery, outcome for the mother and infant were good if the inciting pathology was promptly recognized and treated [8,47–53]. Delay in diagnosis may result in maternal or fetal demise [47,48]. A multidisciplinary approach is critical to a good outcome.

Cesarean sections, wound closure, and complications

Cesarean deliveries occur more frequently in all of the reports of pregnancies after bariatric surgery when compared with the general population. Prior bariatric surgery has been shown to be an independent risk factor [30]. There is not a known physiologic reason for performing more cesarean deliveries among patients who have had bariatric surgery. The increased cesarean rate may be attributed primarily to obstetrician bias or preference. Some obstetricians may prefer to perform an elective cesarean section due to the preconceived notions of increased vaginal delivery risk, and conversion to an emergent cesarean section may be complicated by adhesions from a previous intra-abdominal procedure and by the patient's body habitus (if the patient remains obese). In other instances, the patient may prefer this mode of delivery. An objective evaluation of the benefits and risks of the performance of cesarean delivery in these patients is needed to make an informed recommendation regarding the preferred mode of delivery.

Choosing the optimal incision is crucial when performing cesarean sections in this patient population. The advantages and disadvantages of incision location should be taken into consideration. The type of incision is dependent on the physician comfort level, patient body habitus, and the circumstances surrounding the cesarean delivery. In addition, obesity is a major risk factor for postcesarean wound complications, particularly infection, separation, and dehiscence [54].

In our series, 1 of 15 patients undergoing bariatric surgery (6.7%) experienced a wound-related complication. Our practice routinely uses a Pfannenstiel incision with subcutaneous layer closure only for observed "dead space"; if subcutaneous tissue is opposed, no additional sutures are placed. Staples are routinely used and left in place for 5 to 7 days.

Table 4
Surgical complications in pregnancies following weight loss surgery

Author	Weight loss procedure	Patient age (yr)	Interval from surgery to conception	Fetal EGA (wk)	Complication	Intervention	Outcome
Ramirez and Turrentine [50]	VBG	28	4 yr	26	GIB, band erosion; placental abruption	Laparotomy, band removal; emergency CS	No further complications
Erez et al [51]	LGB	27	2 yr	35	Acute gastric ulcer perforation	Laparotomy, ulcer repair; emergency CS	No further complications
Moore et al [47]	RYGB	41	18 mo	31	IH, SBO	Laparotomy, small bowel resection; emergency CS	Maternal and fetal death
Charles et al [48]	RYGB	23	6 mo	25	IH, SBO	Laparotomy, small bowel resection; vaginal delivery	No further complications
Kakarla et al [8]	RYGB	33	30 mo	13	IH, intermittent SBO	Laparoscopy, reduction, and repair of IH	No further complications
	RYGB	35	9 mo	34	IH, SBO	Laparotomy, reduction, and repair of IH; CS, BTL	Maternal DVT and endometritis, viable infant
Baker and Kothari [52]	RYGB	33	4 mo	25	IH, SBO	Laparotomy, reduction, and repair of IH; CS, BTL	No further complications
Bellanger et al [53]	RYGB	25	2 yr	33	IH, SBO	Laparotomy, reduction, and repair of IH; CS, BTL	No further complications
Ahmed and O'Malley [49]	RYGB	26	8 mo	30	IH, SBO	Laparoscopy, reduction, and repair of IH	No further complications

Abbreviations: BTL, bilateral tubal ligation; CS, cesarean section; EGA, estimated gestational age; GIB, gastrointestinal bleed; IH, internal hernia; LGB, laparoscopic gastric banding; RYGB, Roux-en-Y gastric bypass; SBO, small bowel obstruction; VBG, vertical banded gastroplasty.

Improvement of infertility and polycystic ovarian syndrome

Obesity is associated with infertility. Although the mechanism that causes infertility is not fully understood, it has been postulated that sex hormone–binding globins, androgens, insulin secretion, and resistance have a role [55–58]. Even modest weight loss has been shown to improve fertility [14,55]. Improvements in fertility after weight loss surgery have been shown and seem to be mediated through improved hormonal regulation [14,28,31, 41,55].

Polycystic ovarian syndrome (PCOS) is a complex metabolic abnormality that is not completely understood. The clinical manifestations of this condition include menstrual dysfunction, infertility, high risk of miscarriage, and hyperinsulinemia. There is also an increased risk for endometrial cancer, coronary artery disease, type II diabetes, and stroke [59]. Obesity has been implicated as a key factor in the pathogenesis of PCOS, and weight loss has been shown to ameliorate the constellation of symptoms. Unfortunately, the unsustained results of nonsurgical weight loss often lead to incomplete resolution of symptoms [60].

The effects of bariatric surgery on patients who have PCOS have been investigated. Eid and colleagues [61] retrospectively reviewed the charts of 24 patients who had PCOS and who had undergone a gastric bypass. With a mean follow-up of 27.5 ± 16 months, most patients were noted to have vast improvements or resolution of their preoperative symptoms. All patients had resolution of their menstrual irregularities and dysfunction, and all patients seeking to become pregnant were able to do so without the need for clomiphene. Similarly, Escobar-Morreale and colleagues [62] prospectively followed 12 similar patients and observed recovery of regular and ovulatory menstrual cycles and improvement in insulin resistance in all subjects. This study noted the markedly increased prevalence (6 to 7 fold) of PCOS in the morbidly obese population compared with control subjects. In many of their patients, the syndrome was previously undiagnosed.

These findings provide some physiologic evidence for the observed improvement of fertility after bariatric surgery. Weight loss can decrease menstrual irregularities, achieve a more constant ovulatory pattern, and improve fertility [63,64]. This phenomenon was noted in several studies where previously infertile patients were able to conceive after bariatric surgery [28,31,41]. Although we do not feel that treating PCOS or infertility is an indication for bariatric surgery, this may be considered a significant secondary gain for prospective patients.

Contraception

A great effort has been made in the bariatric literature to recommend delaying pregnancy after bariatric surgery for 18 to 24 months. This may be a difficult task for the patient for many reasons. First, excess weight loss leads to improved fertility as a result of hormonal changes. Second, weight loss may lead to increased sexual activity and libido [28]. Third, oral contraceptive pills, the most widely used form of contraception, may be unreliable after a bariatric procedure [55,65,66].

There is no consensus on the optimal mode of contraception after bariatric surgery. Decreased efficacy of oral contraceptive pills after malabsorptive procedures has been shown after biliopancreatic diversion and jejunoileal bypass [55,67]. Complete efficacy has not been shown and should not be expected after RYGB. The transdermal contraceptive patch has a decreased efficacy in patients who weigh more than 90 kg [68]. Intramuscular depot medroxyprogesterone injections may reliable in this population. Barrier intrauterine contraceptive devices and condoms should remain effective after bariatric surgery. Caution must be used with the diaphragm if the patient has gained or lost 10 to 20 pounds since the diaphragm was fit. It is our preference to recommend medroxyprogesterone, intrauterine contraceptive devices, and condoms.

Summary

Obesity is a modern-day epidemic that can be successfully treated with bariatric surgery. A large proportion of the patients who undergo this procedure yearly are young women. Maternal and fetal outcomes in pregnancies after bariatric surgery are good and do not increase the rate of complications according to several recent studies. It is generally recommended to delay pregnancy for up to 2 years after bariatric surgery; this may be difficult because a consensus on contraception is unavailable in this patient population. This delay should theoretically decrease any nutrition-related complications. Although perinatal care ought to be in the setting of an experienced, multidisciplinary institution, it is our finding that an intense regimen of follow-up and testing may not be warranted. Complications from the bariatric procedure may occur months to years after the procedure and thus should always be considered in the setting of abdominal pain and nausea. Delay in diagnosis of a surgical abdomen can lead to poor outcome. The sustained weight loss from bariatric surgery can "treat" PCOS and infertility. In conclusion, pregnancy after weight loss surgery is safe and has good outcomes.

References

[1] Lara MD, Kothari SN, Sugerman HJ. Surgical management of obesity: a review of the evidence relating health benefits to risks. Treat Endocrinol 2005;4:55–64.

[2] Buchwald H, Avidor Y, Braunwald E, et al. Bariatric surgery: a systematic review and meta-analysis. JAMA 2004;292:1724–37.

[3] Gastrointestinal surgery for severe obesity: National Institutes of Health Consensus Development Conference Statement. Am J Clin Nutr 1992;55:615S–9S.

[4] Brolin RE. Update: NIH consensus conference. Gastrointestinal surgery for severe obesity. Nutrition 1996;12:403–4.

[5] Gastrointestinal surgery for severe obesity. National Institutes of Health Consensus. Conference draft statement on gastrointestinal surgery for severe obesity. Obes Surg 1991;1(3): 257–65.

[6] Flegal KM, Carroll MD, Ogden CL, et al. Prevalence and trends in obesity among U.S. adults, 1999–2000. JAMA 2002;288:1723–7.

[7] Pope GD, Birkmeyer JD, Finlayson SR. National trends in utilization and in-hospital outcomes of bariatric surgery. J Gastrointest Surg 2002;6:855–60.

[8] Kakarla N, Dailey C, Marino T, et al. Pregnancy after gastric bypass surgery and internal hernia formation. Obstet Gynecol 2005;105:1195–8.

[9] Weiss JL, Malone FD, Emig D, et al. Obesity, obstetric complications and cesarean delivery rate: a population-based screening study. Am J Obstet Gynecol 2004;190(4): 1091–7.

[10] Naeye RL. Maternal body weight and pregnancy outcome. Am J Clin Nutr 1990;52:273–9.

[11] Abrams B, Parker J. Overweight and pregnancy complications. Int J Obes 1988;12:293–303.

[12] Hood DD, Dewan DM. Anesthetic and obstetric outcomes in morbidly obese parturients. Anesthesiology 1993;79:1210–9.

[13] Gross T, Sokol RJ, King KC. Obesity in pregnancy: risks and outcome. Obstet Gynecol 1980;56:446–50.

[14] Deitel M, Stone E, Kassam HA, et al. Gynecologic-obstetric changes after loss of massive excess weight following bariatric surgery. J Am Coll Nutr 1988;7:147–53.

[15] Cedergren MI. Maternal obesity and the risk of adverse pregnancy outcome. Obstet Gynecol 2004;103:219–24.

[16] Morin KH. Perinatal outcomes of obese women: a review of the literature. J Obstet Gynecol Neonatal Nurs 1998;27:431–40.

[17] Hey H, Nieburh-Jorgensen U. Jejuno-ileal bypass surgery in obesity: gynecological and obstetrical aspects. Acta Obstet Gynecol Scand 1981;60:135–40.

[18] Taylor JL, O'Leary JP. Pregnancy following jejuno-ileal bypass: effects on fetal outcome. Obstet Gynecol 1976;48:425–7.

[19] Ingardia CJ, Fischer JR. Pregnancy after jejunoileal bypass and SGA infant. Obstet Gynecol 1978;52:215–8.

[20] Knudsen LB, Kallen B. Intestinal bypass operation and pregnancy outcome. Acta Obstet Gynecol Scand 1986;65:831–4.

[21] Haddow JE, Hill LE, Kloza EM, et al. Neural tube defects after gastric bypass. Lancet 1986; 1:1330.

[22] Granstrom L, Backman L. Fetal growth retardation after gastric banding. Acta Obstet Gynecol Scand 1990;69:533–6.

[23] Biron S, Hould F, Simard S. Birthweight after biliopancratic diversion. Obes Surg 1999;9: 126.

[24] Woodard CB. Pregnancy following bariatric surgery. J Perinat Neonatal Nurs 2004;18(4): 329–40.

[25] Malinowski SS. Nutritional and metabolic complications of bariatric surgery. Am J Med Sci 2006;31(4) 219–215.

[26] Alvarez-Leite JI. Nutrient deficiencies secondary to bariatric sugery. Curr Opin Clin Nutr Metab Care 2004;7:569–75.

[27] Skull AJ, Slater GH, Duncombe JE, et al. Laparoscopic adjustable banding in pregnancy: safety, patient tolerance, and effect on obesity-related pregnancy outcomes. Obes Surg 2004;11:230–5.

[28] Marceau P, Kaufman D, Biron S, et al. Outcomes of pregnancies after biliopancreatic diversion. Obes Surg 2004;14:318–24.

[29] Dixon JB, Dixon ME, O'Brien PE. Birth outcomes in obese women after laparoscopic adjustable gastric banding. Obstet Gynecol 2005;106:965–72.

[30] Sheiner E, Levy A, Silverberg D, et al. Pregnancy after bariatric surgery is not associated with adverse perinatal outcome. Am J Obstet Gynecol 2004;190:1335–40.

[31] Friedman J, Cuneo S, Valenzano M, et al. Pregnancies in an 18-year follow-up after biliopancreatic diversion. Obes Surg 1995;5:308–13.

[32] Wittgrove AC, Jester L, Wittgrove P, et al. Pregnancy following gastric bypass for morbid obesity. Obes Surg 1998;8:461–4.

[33] Bar-Zohar D, Azem F, Klausner J, et al. Pregnancy after laparosopic adjustable banding: perinatal outcome is favorable also for women with relatively high gestational weight gain. Surg Endosc 2006;20:1580–3.

[34] Rand CSW, Macgregor AMC. Medical care and pregnancy outcome after gastric bypass surgery for obesity. South Med J 1989;10:1319–20.

[35] Richards DS, Miler DK, Goodman GN. Pregnancy after gastric bypass for morbid obesity. J Reprod Med 1987;32(3):172–6.

[36] Bilenka B, Ben-Shlomo I, Cozacov C, et al. Fertility, miscarriage and pregnancy after vertical banded gastroplasty operation for morbid obesity. Acta Obstet Gynecol Scand 1995;74: 42–4.

[37] Weiss HG, Nehoda H, Labeck B, et al. Pregnancies after adjustable gastric banding. Obes Surg 2001;11:303–6.

[38] Michlin R, Oettinger M, Odeh M, et al. Maternal obesity and pregnancy outcome. Isr Med Assoc J 2001;2(1):10–3.

[39] Perlow JH, Morgan MA, Montgomery D, et al. Perinatal outcome in pregnancy complicated by massive obesity. Am J Obstet Gynecol 1992;167:958–62.

[40] Grossetti E, Beucher G, Regeasse A, et al. Obstetrical complications in morbid obesity. J Gynecol Obstet Biol Reprod (Paris) 2004;33(8):739–44.

[41] Dixon JB, Dixon ME, O'Brien PR. Pregnancy after Lap-Band surgery: management of the band to achieve healthy weight outcomes. Obese Surg 2001;11:59–65.

[42] Garza E, Kuhn J, Arnold D, et al. Internal hernias after laparoscopic Roux-en-Y gastric bypass. Am J Surg 2004;188:796–800.

[43] Higa KD, Ho T, Boon KB. Internal hernia after laparoscopic Roux-en-Y gastric bypass: incidence, treatment, and prevention. Obes Surg 2003;13:350–4.

[44] Cucchiaro G, Rossitch JC, Bowie J, et al. Clinical significance of ultrasonographically detected coincidental gallstones. Dig Dis Sci 1990;35(4):417–21.

[45] Blachar A, Federle MP, Brancatelli G, et al. Radiologist performance in the diagnosis of internal hernia by using specific CT findings with emphasis on transmesenteric hernia. Radiology 2001;221:422–8.

[46] Eckhauser A, Torquati A, Youssef Y, et al. Internal hernia: postoperative complication of Roux-en-Y gastric bypass surgery. Am Surg 2006;72(7):581–5.

[47] Moore KA, Ouyang DW, Whang EE. Maternal and fetal deaths after gastric bypass surgery for morbid obesity. N Engl J Med 2004;351(7):721–2.

[48] Charles A, Domingo S, Goldfadden A, et al. Small bowel ischemia after Roux-en-Y gastric bypass complicated by pregnancy: a case report. Am Surg 2005;71(3):231–4.

[49] Ahmed AR, O'Malley W. Internal hernia with Roux loop obstruction during pregnancy after gastric bypass surgery. Obes Surg 2006;16:1246–8.

[50] Ramirez MM, Turrentine MA. Gastrointestinal hemorrhage during pregnancy in a patient with a history of vertical-banded gastroplasty. Am J Obstet Gynecol 1995;173:1630–1.

[51] Erez O, Maymon E, Mazor M. Acute gastric ulcer perforation in a 35 weeks' nulliparous patient with gastric banding. Am J Obstet Gynecol 2004;191:1721–2.

[52] Baker MT, Kothari SN. Successful surgical treatment of a pregnancy-induced Petersen's hernia after laparoscopic gastric bypass. Surg Obes Relat Dis 2005;1:506–8.

[53] Bellanger DE, Ruiz JF, Solar K. Small bowel obstruction complicating pregnancy after laparoscopic gastric bypass. Surg Obes Relat Dis 2006;2:490–2.

[54] Vermillion ST, Lamoutte C, Soper DE, et al. Wound infection after cesarean: effect of subcutaneous tissue thickness. Obstet Gynecol 2000;95:923–6.

528 PATEL et al

[55] Gerrits EG, Ceulemans R, van Hee R, et al. Contraceptive treatment after biliopancreatic diversion needs consensus. Obes Surg 2003;13:378–82.
[56] Crosignani PG, Colombo M, Vegetti W, et al. Overweight and obese anovulatory patients with polycystic ovaries: parallel improvements in anthropometric indices, ovarian physiology and fertility rate induced by diet. Hum Reprod 2003;18(9):1928–32.
[57] Barbieri RL, Smith S, Ryan KJ. The role of hyperinsulinemia in the pathogenesis of ovarian hyperandrogenism. Fertil Steril 1988;38:406–9.
[58] Kiddy DS, Sharp PS, White DM, et al. Differences in clinical and endocrine features between obese and non obese subjects with polycystic ovarian syndrome: an analysis of 263 consecutive cases. Clin Endocrinol 1990;32:213–20.
[59] Carr BR. Disorders of the ovaries and female reproductive tract. In: Williams RH, editor. Williams' textbook of endocrinology. Philadelphia: WB Saunders; 1998. p. 787–90.
[60] Asuncion M, Calvo RM, San Millan JL, et al. A prospective study of the prevalence of polycystic ovary syndrome is unselected Caucasian women from Spain. J Clin Endocrinol Metab 2000;85 2434–8.
[61] Eid GM, Cottam DR, Velcu LM, et al. Effective treatment of polycystic ovarian syndrome with Roux-en-Y gastric bypass. Surg Obes Relat Dis 2005;1:77–80.
[62] Escobar-Morreale HF, Botella-Carretero JI, Alvarez-Blasco F, et al. The polycystic ovarian syndrome associated with morbid obesity may resolve after weight loss induced by bariatric surgery. J Clin Endocrinol Metab 2005;90:6364–9.
[63] Bastounis EA, Karayiannakis AJ, Syrigos K, et al. Sex hormone changes in morbidly obese patients after vertical banded gastroplasty. Eur Surg Res 1998;30:43–7.
[64] Davies MJ. Evidence for effects of weight on reproduction in women. Reprod Biomed Online 2006;12(5):552–61.
[65] Deitel M, Ternamian AM. Gynecologic-obstetric features of morbid obesity and the effect of weight loss. In: Deitel M, editor. Update: surgery for the morbidly obese patient. Toronto: FD-Communications Inc; 2000. p. 481–5.
[66] Deitel M. Pregnancy after bariatric surgery. Obes Surg 1998;8:465–6.
[67] Johansson ED, Krai JG. Oral contraceptives after intestinal bypass operations. JAMA 1976; 236(25):2847.
[68] Courtney C. The contraceptive patch: latest developments. AWHONN Lifelines 2006;10(3): 250–4.

ELSEVIER
SAUNDERS

Med Clin N Am 91 (2007) 529–536

THE MEDICAL
CLINICS
OF NORTH AMERICA

Index

Note: Page numbers of article titles are in **boldface** type.

A

Abdominal pain
    after gastric bypass, 472–476
    in pregnancy, 521–522

Adhesions, 475–476

Adipokines
    bariatric surgery effects on, 425–426
    in insulin resistance, 396–397

Adiponectin
    bariatric surgery effects on, 425–426
    in insulin resistance, 397

Adipose cells, insulin resistance and,
    396–397

Adjustable gastric banding (AGB)
    band adjustment in, 520–521
    effectiveness of, 326–328
    insurance coverage of, 335
    laparoscopic. *See* Laparoscopic
        adjustable gastric banding
        (LAGB).

Adolescents, bariatric surgery for, 383–384,
    386

AGB. *See* Adjustable gastric banding
    (AGB).

Anemia, after bariatric surgery, 387

Anesthesia
    intraoperative management of, 348
    preoperative evaluation for, 347
    pulmonary considerations in, 436

Anxiety disorders, 451–454

Appetite control, postoperative, 457

Asthma
    bariatric surgery effects on, 439
    in obesity, 434–435

Atherosclerosis
    bariatric surgery effects on, 421
    in insulin resistance syndrome, 398
    in polycystic ovary syndrome, 402

Atrial fibrillation, in obesity, 418

B

Banding, gastric, adjustable. *See* Adjustable
    gastric banding (AGB).

Bariatric surgery
    body contouring after, 463
    cardiovascular disease and, **415–431**
    cholecystectomy with, 445–447
    complications of. *See* Complications.
    contraindications for, 340–341
    cost-effectiveness of, 330–333
    costs of, 329–330
    diabetes mellitus management after,
        407–408
    eating disorders before and after,
        454–458
    effectiveness of, 326–329
    for challenging patients, **383–392**
        adolescents, 383–384, 386
        elderly, 385, 388–389
        pregnant, 387–388
        super obese, 384–385, 389–390
    for metabolic disorders, 402–409
    gastrointestinal disorders after,
        443–450
    guidelines for, 335–336
    indications for, 326–329
    insurance coverage for, 334–335
    laparoscopic. *See* Laparoscopic
        procedures; *subjects starting with*
        Laparoscopic.
    mortality rate in. *See* Mortality rate.
    nutrition after. *See* Nutritional
        consequences.
    nutritionist role in, 341–342
    options for, 326–329
    outcome of
        pulmonary, 438–439
        versus volume of procedures,
            370–375
    perioperative care in, **339–351**
    pregnancy after, **515–528**
    primer on, **353–381**
    procedures for. *See also individual*
        procedures.
        selection of, 359–370
        types of, 326, 357–358

INDEX

T

Thromboembolism, 345, 437–438, 478–479

U

Ulceration, marginal, after gastric bypass, 474–475

Ursodeoxycholic acid, for gallstone dissolution, 446–447

V

VBG. *See* Vertical banded gastroplasty (VBG).

Venothromboembolism
  postoperative, 437–438, 478–479
  preoperative screening for, 345

Ventricular ectopy, in obesity, 418

Vertical banded gastroplasty (VBG)
  cardiovascular effects of, 424
  eating behavior modification after, 508–509
  effectiveness of, 326–329
  failure of, 357–358
  pregnancy after, 518

Vitamin(s)
  deficiencies of

after bariatric surgery, 387, 477, 479
after LRYGB procedure, 366–367
preoperative, 503–504
metabolism of, 501–502
supplementation of, 510–511

Volvulus, 475–476

Vomiting. *See* Nausea and vomiting.

W

Weight loss
  excessive, after gastric banding, 495
  inadequate, after gastric banding, 494–495
  postoperative, binge eating and, 456–457
  suboptimal, 461–462, 479–480

Wernicke's polyneuropathy, 479

Wound complications, 356–357, 480–481, 522

Z

Zinc
  deficiency of, 479
  supplementation of, 510

Moving?

Make sure your subscription moves with you!

To notify us of your new address, find your **Clinics Account Number** (located on your mailing label above your name), and contact customer service at:

E-mail: elspcs@elsevier.com

800-654-2452 (subscribers in the U.S. & Canada)
407-345-4000 (subscribers outside of the U.S. & Canada)

Fax number: 407-363-9661

Elsevier Periodicals Customer Service
6277 Sea Harbor Drive
Orlando, FL 32887-4800

*To ensure uninterrupted delivery of your subscription, please notify us at least 4 weeks in advance of move.

ELSEVIER